Praise for
THE POWER WE HOLD

'This book is dangerous – in the best way possible. Isabella exposes the systems that have kept women's bodies misunderstood and misdiagnosed for generations, and she does it with unapologetic brilliance. The Power We Hold *is equal parts science, rage, and reclamation. Every woman who's ever been dismissed, disbelieved, or gaslit by medicine needs this book like oxygen.'*

DR. JOLENE BRIGHTEN, FABNE, MSCP, AUTHOR OF *IS THIS NORMAL?*

'Finally, a book all women have been waiting for and need. The Power We Hold *confronts the lies, silencing, and gaslighting that have separated us from our deepest truth. Isabella Mainwaring hands us back our authority — the voice of intuition, the wisdom of spirit, and the power we hold within. As someone who has spent a lifetime awakening intuition around the world, I can say with certainty: this book is bold, liberating, and essential for every woman ready to rise.'*

SONIA CHOQUETTE, BEST-SELLING AUTHOR OF *ASK YOUR GUIDES*

'I cried tears of relief reading this book. For so long "women's issues" have been relegated to our biology and psychology being inferior. Women have been led to believe that their difficulties are self-inflicted. The Power We Hold *shatters this illusion one chapter at a time. Isabella Mainwaring skillfully identifies the systems that oppress women's power AND the science and soul that has the capacity to liberate women's power. The world needs this book.'*

TAMU THOMAS, AUTHOR OF *WOMEN WHO WORK TOO MUCH*

'This book holds the code to return safely back to your power. A power resting in the body that Isabella, scientifically, holistically, and humanly, justifies has long been withheld, mistrusted, and denied. It is not just an instruction to follow, but a life-changing alarm bell for women to shift from surviving to thriving, with our health not failing as a consequence but being the very key through which we unlock our fullest potential. This book is a deep calling, which belongs firmly on the bedside table of the women who are ready to rise and reconstruct a better life, for today, tomorrow, and our collective future.'

HENIKA PATEL, FOUNDER OF THE SCHOOL OF SENSUAL ARTS AND AUTHOR OF *SENSUAL*

'The Power We Hold *is a seismic reclamation. Isabella Mainwaring doesn't just speak truth, she embodies it, offering a rare transmission that fuses science, somatics, and soul. This book will rewire your understanding of power, pleasure, and the intelligence of your own body. It's the missing link for every high-performing woman who's done all the "right" things but still feels disconnected, burnt out, or betrayed by her biology. Isabella reminds us that we're not broken – we've just been living in systems that gaslight our brilliance. Her Root Restoration Framework is a quiet revolution, one that doesn't demand obedience from the body, but invites it home to safety, aliveness, and power. Read this fierce, poetic reclamation of the body's brilliance, and let it change everything.'

VICTORIA SONG, *WALL STREET JOURNAL* BEST-SELLING AUTHOR OF *BENDING REALITY*

THE POWER HOLD

THE POWER HOLD

Reclaiming Our Health from a System That Fails Women

Isabella Mainwaring

HAY HOUSE

Carlsbad, California • New York City
London • Sydney • New Delhi

Published in the United Kingdom by:
Hay House UK Ltd, 1st Floor, Crawford Corner,
91–93 Baker Street, London W1U 6QQ
Tel: +44 (0)20 3927 7290; www.hayhouse.co.uk

Text © Isabella Mainwaring, 2025

Interior illustrations: 56, 75, 126, 131, 178 © Isabella Mainwaring

The moral rights of the author have been asserted.

All rights reserved. No part of this book may be reproduced by any mechanical, photographic or electronic process, or in the form of a phonographic recording; nor may it be stored in a retrieval system, transmitted or otherwise be copied for public or private use, other than for 'fair use' as brief quotations embodied in articles and reviews, without prior written permission of the publisher.

The information given in this book should not be treated as a substitute for professional medical advice; always consult a medical practitioner. Any use of information in this book is at the reader's discretion and risk. Neither the author nor the publisher can be held responsible for any loss, claim or damage arising out of the use, or misuse, of the suggestions made, the failure to take medical advice or for any material on third-party websites.

A catalogue record for this book is available from the British Library.

Tradepaper ISBN: 978-1-83782-464-9
E-book ISBN: 978-1-83782-467-0
Audiobook ISBN: 978-1-83782-465-6

10 9 8 7 6 5 4 3 2 1

This product uses responsibly sourced papers, including recycled materials and materials from other controlled sources. For more information, see www.hayhouse.co.uk

The authorized representative in the EU for product safety and compliance is Penguin Random House Ireland, Morrison Chambers, 32 Nassau Street, Dublin D02 YH68, Ireland. https://eu-contact.penguin.ie

Printed and bound by CPI Group (UK) Ltd, Croydon CR0 4YY

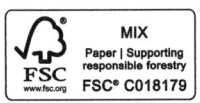

For the women who came before me – the healers, the wild ones, the truth-tellers who dared to trust their bodies and own their power – you're not forgotten.

Your legacy lives in every page of this book.

For the women yet to come – may you remember what the world tried to make you forget:
Your body reflects the balance of the society you live in.
Your reproductive cycle isn't a burden. It's a blueprint.
Your emotions are an ancient wisdom.
Your symptoms are not flaws – they're signals.
Guiding you back to your power.

CONTENTS

Author's Note	xv
Introduction	xix

PART I: YOU'RE NOT BROKEN – THE SYSTEM IS

Chapter 1:	**Rediscovering Lost Wisdom**	**3**
	The Female Edge	4
	How Women's Power Was Erased from History	5
	From Sacred to Sinful: The Dawn of Patriarchy	10
	From Midwives to the Margins	13
	The New Frontier: Reproductive Rights	15
Chapter 2:	**How Patriarchy Shaped Modern Medicine**	**17**
	Men as the Human Standard	18
	Our Health Is Relational	20
	The Myth of Genetic Destiny	22
	The Missing Piece of the Medical Puzzle	23
Chapter 3:	**Imposter Syndrome or Imposter Systems?**	**25**
	Masculine and Feminine: Complementary Energies	26
	How Patriarchy Perpetuates Itself	27

When Women Become Agents of Patriarchy	31
Tracing the Roots of Our Disconnection	33

Chapter 4: Women as an Indicator Species — 37

Signals, Not Symptoms	38
Women's Biological Brilliance	40
We Aren't Defective, We're Responsive	41
Our Bodies Are Barometers of Balance	42

Chapter 5: The Biology Lesson That Women Deserve — 45

Hormones: Our Body's Messengers	46
The Hormone Hierarchy	47
Tier 1 Hormones: The Foundational Regulators	47
Tier 2 Hormones: The Builders	48
Tier 3 Hormones: The Specialists	48
What Are Your Hormones Telling You?	49

Chapter 6: A 'Superior' Biological Blueprint — 53

Our Cyclical Rhythms	54
Daily and Monthly Cycles: Men vs. Women	55
Seasonal Cycles	57
Life Cycles	58
Generational Cycles	60

Chapter 7: It's Time for Gender Equity — 63

From Equality to Equity	64
Power Was Never Outside of You	66
The Sanctuary of Safety	68

Chapter 8: Introducing the Root Restoration Framework — 71

Reclaiming Our Inner Safety and Power	72
The Root Restoration Framework and ThetaSomatics™	73

Uncovering the Root Cause of Your Symptoms	75
From Holding It All to Holding Yourself	79

PART II: THE SYSTEM IN YOUR CELLS

Chapter 9: Stress Is More Than What We've Been Told	**83**
The Real Definition of Stress	84
Our Allostatic Load (Stress Bucket)	85
Understanding the Stress Response	86
The Body-Wide Effects of Stress	89
Completing the 'Stress Response Cycle'	90
Chapter 10: Unlocking the Secrets of the Female Nervous System	**93**
The Nervous System 101	94
Female vs Male Nervous System	101
Oxytocin: Sustainer of Life	102
The Impact of the Menstrual Cycle	104
Chapter 11: The Trauma We Don't See	**109**
The Silent Scripts We Live By	110
Attachment and Authenticity	112
The Trauma Spectrum	114
The Nuances of Female Trauma	117
Your Body Is an Archive	118
Chapter 12: Rewiring Our Wounds	**123**
How Survival Gets Wired into the Body	124
The Survival Loop	125
Interrupting the Survival Loop	130
Your Triggers Are Clues	132

Chapter 13: The Adaptive Self vs The Authentic Self	**135**
Shame: A Cultural Weapon	136
Reclaiming Our Voice	140
Our Power Pipeline: The Womb–Throat Axis	141
Breaking Free of Obedience	148
Angry Women	149
Express, Don't Explain, Yourself	151
Chapter 14: Machines Regulate, Humans Feel	**153**
What Are Emotions, Exactly?	154
Neuropeptides: 'Molecules of Emotion'	156
The Implications of Unexpressed Emotions	158
How Suppressed Emotions Impact Our Health	161
You Have to Feel It to Heal It	165
Emotional Sensitivity: Women's Superpower	167
Chapter 15: Women – from Indicators to Initiators	**169**
A Force of Nurture	170
Building the New System	171

PART III: RISING FROM THE ROOT

Chapter 16: Root Restoration: Creating Mind and Body Safety	**177**
The Five Core Roots of Safety	177
How to Approach Root Restoration	179
Trust Your Timeline	181
Chapter 17: Root 1: Authenticity	**183**
Feeling Safe to Be You	184
Getting to the Core of Who You Are	185
The Authenticity Audit	186
Daily Practice: Authenticity in Action	189

Chapter 18: Root 2: Conscious Safety	191
The Life Audit	191
Daily Practice: Conscious Safety in Action	194
Chapter 19: Root 3: Environmental Safety	197
Getting Back to Basics	198
Daily Practice: Back to Basics in Action	203
Prioritizing Pleasure	204
Daily Practice: Embrace Pleasure	205
Aligning with Your Biological Blueprint	206
Chapter 20: Root 4: Historical Safety	213
Cultivating Historical Safety	214
Phase 1: Release the Old	215
Phase 2: Regulate to Rewire	225
Ending the Survival Loop	227
Chapter 21: Root 5: Unconscious Safety	231
Confronting Our Beliefs and Patterns	232
Cultivating Unconscious Safety	233
Step 1: Become Aware of Your Adaptive Beliefs	233
Step 2: Show Your Subconscious That Your Authentic Beliefs Are Safe	237
Step 3: ThetaSomatics™ Rewiring Practice	241
Daily Practice: Act from Your Authentic Belief	247
How to Recognize Signs of Rewiring	248
Conclusion	253
References	257
Acknowledgments	269
About the Author	273

AUTHOR'S NOTE

This book is a love letter to women and a call to reclaim the power we've always held. A power that was revered for most of human history but has been systematically obscured, diminished, even erased, by millennia of biological, psychological, and social forces under patriarchy.

From medical gaslighting to emotional suppression, and from environmental toxins to the constant hum of comparison culture, these forces have quietly rewritten the way we see ourselves, the way we care for ourselves – especially our reproductive health – and the way we interpret the signals our bodies send us every single day.

But this isn't just a women's issue – it's a human issue that reflects deeper imbalances within our culture. Our patriarchal social blueprint has been designed to corrode the well-being of those outside its center – which includes women and those who exist beyond the modern male/female gender binary. In this book, my goal is to illuminate these patterns; not to point fingers but to spark awareness, inspire transformation, and advocate for meaningful change.

As women, this is our moment. We're standing on the threshold of Pluto's return to Aquarius, and the last time that happened, the world underwent a period of explosive transformation: the French, American, and Haitian revolutions; the collapse of monarchies and feudal systems; and the birth of the Declaration of Human Rights.

All this unfolded within just two decades (1778 to 1798) – each moment a rebellion, a reckoning, a breaking point where the old order couldn't contain the rising tide of the new. And the American psychological astrologer Dr. Jennifer Freed reminds us that we're entering that archetypal terrain again – a time when systems crack and new structures rise.

Aquarius doesn't follow rules – it rewrites them. It urges us to dismantle outdated models and reimagine the future. Gender roles, relationship structures, the meaning of work and success, our connection with technology, and even the systems that govern our lives – between now and 2044, all are up for radical reinvention.

Astrology isn't a belief system – it's the world's oldest language of cycles, rooted in math and observation. And as history shows, revolutionary cycles repeat. The words 'revolution' and 'revolve' were born from the Latin word *revolvere*, meaning to roll back or turn again. A reminder that revolutions aren't just eruptions, they're returns.

And we're in the midst of one now. The old systems are crumbling, and the future demands new leaders: women who embody both strength and softness; women who lead not through dominance, pushing, and forcing but through deep connection, intuition, and creation. The future of humanity and our planet requires that women step into their full power and potential.

• • •

I come from an upper-middle-class family and attended schools and universities in the UK and Australia – two Western, patriarchal societies – so I'm a product of the environment in which I grew up and learned about the world. As a cisgender white woman who identifies with those categories and having two heterosexual parents who are still very happily married, my experience with gender and sex identities has been straightforward.

However, I recognize that for many, the language available to define their identities can feel insufficient, restraining, or exclusionary. So, in this book, I use the words woman, women, and we, as well as man, men, and they, to describe biological and social experiences tied to female biology, along with the broader experiences associated with these identities.

Throughout, I've done my best to interrogate women's past, present, and future through the eyes of as many women as possible, but I don't assume that I speak for all of us. And of course, I acknowledge that not all individuals who menstruate, experience pregnancy, or face reproductive health challenges identify as women.

I've tried to explore these topics with respect and compassion for diverse identities, while focusing on patterns I've identified that are rooted in physiology and psychology. I believe that by understanding how our behavior and health are shaped by multigenerational dynamics, environmental pressures, and social contexts, we can move away from assigning blame and open the door to personal responsibility and collective empowerment.

While describing events from my own past or relaying the stories of some of my clients, I've leaned on family, friends, and the women I've worked with to fact-check my words. Of course, this book is written from my lived experience, and as such it's not a definitive account but one voice in a much larger story.

To protect client identities, I've changed some details and anonymized names on request. In some cases, composite characters have been created to further protect privacy while still conveying the essence of the person's experience. I'm deeply grateful to the women who have entrusted me with their stories – shared with courage, clarity, and vulnerability – and my aim is to present them accurately and respectfully, ensuring the confidentiality and trust of those who have shared their lives with me.

INTRODUCTION

*'Our deepest fear is not that
we are inadequate. [It's] that we are
powerful beyond measure.'*

MARIANNE WILLIAMSON

We say we want empowerment. But what most women are practicing, day in and day out, isn't empowerment – it's endurance. And it's costing us everything. This realization hit me like a punch to the gut as I sat in a conference room filled with women CEOs, thought leaders, entrepreneurs, scientists, and celebrities at the annual meeting of the World Economic Forum in Davos, Switzerland, in January 2020.

I was just 22 years old and believed that attending this invitation-only brunch on feminine leadership alongside my boss would be the pinnacle of my career. But something felt deeply off. As I listened to each woman's polished introduction and visionary ideas, I couldn't ignore what was simmering beneath the surface – the depletion in their voices, the fatigue in their eyes, the strain wrapped in perfectly curated poise.

These leaders had shattered glass ceilings and claimed seats at the world's most exclusive tables, but their bodies were quietly breaking under the weight of it all. Burnout, perfectionism, miscarriages, loneliness, anxiety, infertility, autoimmune disease, and hormone imbalances were woven through *every* story. These women had succeeded by every metric that society celebrates, but it had come at a price.

A Moment of Reckoning

On the second night of the forum, my own body began to revolt. I was staying in a large expedition tent pitched in the snow, just 20 meters from a luxury hotel. By day, the tent served as a hub for educating world leaders about the climate crisis. By night, it transformed into a dormitory, lined with sleeping bags and filled with the soft murmurs of breath.

When I arrived back at the tent around midnight, the lights were out. I slipped through the entrance, careful not to let in the cold air. Dozens of bodies lay curled in sleep, and I used the soft glow of my cell phone to guide me. Every rustle of my coat felt loud. Every step felt intrusive. Eventually, I found a narrow space between two strangers and slid into it slowly, unzipping my bag quietly to avoid waking anyone.

As soon as I settled, the pain began. Sharp waves of period cramps washing over me. Mortified, I lay still, jaw clenched, willing myself to stay quiet. I didn't groan. I didn't shift. I didn't dare get up so that I could trudge through the snow to the hotel in search of pain relief.

But as the tears streamed down my face and the cramps pulsed through me, a veil lifted, and suddenly, I could see how deeply I'd been conditioned to ignore my body's needs. How instinctively I'd learned to minimize my suffering, to make myself small, to endure discomfort without making a sound, even in the most primal expressions of my humanity. This quiet tyranny of self-silencing that I'd carried for so long was fully illuminated.

As I lay there, I recalled the stories of endurance told by the women around that brunch table and I couldn't help but wonder: *What if women have been taught to chase success in a system that wasn't designed with us in mind? In a world that asks us to abandon our bodies in order to belong?*

The Cost of Playing by the 'Rules'

Ongoing research reveals that the so-called personality traits commonly seen in people who suffer from chronic illness (and, I'd argue, reproductive health issues) are in fact the behaviors that we demand from women.

Among them is an automatic and compulsive concern for the emotional needs of others and ignoring one's own. As Elise Loehnen, author of *On Our Best Behaviour: The Price Women Pay to be Good*, so precisely put it: 'Women are conditioned to be good. Men are culturally conditioned for power, programmed for power.'

When I started to look more closely at the interconnected biological, psychological, and social forces that contribute to the health challenges women face, I soon realized that the norms and expectations of patriarchy – our culture's dominant social ideology, which upholds male power through control, suppression, and systemic inequality – are deeply ingrained in them. And after understanding that, I couldn't look back.

As we'll explore in the book, over millennia, patriarchy influenced beliefs and created a worldview: one that prioritized control over compassion, facts over feeling, efficiency over empathy, and productivity over presence. Capitalism, which emerged alongside patriarchy, then scaled those values into systems that became global through colonization.

Entire continents were reorganized around extraction, control, and profit. Cultures that once honored interdependence, cyclical rhythms, and embodied wisdom were systematically dismantled, often violently. Women's roles were recast as secondary. And the wisdom of the body – especially the female body – was deemed irrational, unproductive, or dangerous.

Of course, men also paid a price under patriarchy, but today, they also continue to benefit from a system that privileges them. As *The New York Times* declared during the height of the COVID-19 pandemic, women – especially mothers – are the 'shock absorbers of society.'[1] And true to that description, women are now bearing the brunt of a growing health crisis driven by chronic stress. Women's bodies have a heightened response to stress, so our symptoms are the first to appear – and they are early signals of a much deeper collective breakdown.

And I believe that if we don't radically change the way we approach health and healing, men won't be far behind us. In fact, many already aren't. Men account for 80 percent of suicides in the US[2] – a statistic that's reflected across many Western countries. At the same time, global sperm counts have dropped by more than 50 percent in the last 40 years.[3]

Both issues are symptoms of a deeper crisis that women's bodies have been trying to communicate for centuries. If we continue to ignore them, we'll *all* pass the point of no return.

Your Body Isn't the Problem, It's the Solution

When I first came across research showing that women have an increased sensitivity to stress – both biologically and psychologically – I felt angry. It seemed unfair: another strike against us in a world where we're already fighting to keep up. How are we supposed to 'have it all' – good health, nourishing relationships, and successful careers – if our biology is a disadvantage?

But the more I learned, the more my understanding shifted in the opposite direction. For most of human history, women were revered for their unique ability to perceive and respond to stress, guiding communities back to systems and practices that ensured the survival of our species. I cannot emphasize this enough: Women's heightened ability to sense, feel, and respond to internal and external shifts is an evolutionary advantage, not a weakness.

So, whatever your reason for picking up this book, I celebrate your curiosity and desire to understand how your body works and what it's trying to tell you. For those who are struggling with debilitating symptoms, conditions, or reproductive health issues, as I have, I kept you especially in mind as I wrote it.

And while I've shared insights from the latest advances in Western medicine – alongside wisdom from ancient and Eastern healing traditions – I've also woven in the lived experiences and powerful transformations of real women from around the world. I believe that the most trustworthy and empowering knowledge about women's bodies comes from the integration of what medical science has confirmed in recent decades and the deep, embodied knowing that all women carry within them.

It's my intention to inform, empower, and encourage you because women's bodies *work*, and they *know* how to heal and self-repair when we create the right conditions. Whatever health concerns you're confronted with, now or in the future, the insights you gain from this book will be there to support you. I'll take you from understanding the forces that have shaped your reality, to uncovering how these forces have wired your mind and body, and ultimately, to a process of deep restoration and a reclamation of your power.

How to Use the Book

To receive the full potency of this work, I invite you to move through the book in the order it's presented. You may feel the urge to skip ahead to the healing practices in Part III, especially if you're navigating symptoms right now. But if you bypass the exploration of *why* and *how* these symptoms are occurring in the first place – in Parts I and II – you'll miss the most powerful part of all: the deeper understanding that rewires your relationship with your body and your health.

The inner 'click' that changes how you see yourself, and what you believe is possible. And when that shift comes, successful results become inevitable.

In **Part I, You're Not Broken, the System Is**, you'll uncover how patriarchal systems – including clinical medicine – have shaped society, culture, and even biology, pushing women's bodies to the brink in the process. We'll look at how, over time, these systems have replaced wisdom with control, reverence with repression, and healing with hierarchy.

You'll realize that the struggles you thought were yours alone – your symptoms, your self-doubt, your disconnection – are not evidence of your 'brokenness' but signals that the system is failing.

In **Part II, The System in Your Cells**, we turn inward, to understand how these patriarchal systems have been absorbed into our cells, nervous system, and beliefs. We'll map the science and somatics of stress, trauma, inauthenticity, and survival – exploring how women's chronic symptoms, burnout, hormonal chaos, and emotional suppression are responses to our cultural conditioning.

This is where the shift happens, from 'I need help' to 'I hold the keys.' From 'What's wrong with me?' to 'I know exactly what my body needs – and I'll give it to her.' From outsourcing your health, to owning it.

In **Part III, Rising from the Root**, awareness and understanding turn to action. I'll guide you through the Root Restoration Framework – my practical, step-by-step protocol to free your body's systems from overwhelm, expand the capacity of your nervous system, release stored emotion, reconnect with your authentic self, and restore your body's natural intelligence.

This is where my unique therapeutic method, ThetaSomatics™, enters the picture (somatics is the study and practice of how experiences, emotions, and social conditioning live in the body – and how we can transform them by working through the body). With the help of somatic tools that combine the rewiring of subconscious beliefs, nervous system regulation, emotional release, and the activation of safety-based hormones, you'll begin to walk a new path – one rooted in inner safety and radical self-trust.

• • •

This isn't just a book. It's a reclamation. Woven throughout, you'll find self-reflection practices – invitations to remember, to reconnect. You can keep a journal close as you read, or simply come back to them in your own time.

The word 'heal' comes from the Old English *hælan,* meaning 'to make whole.' This reminds us that healing isn't just about fixing what's broken but about remembering what's always been whole within us.

Part I
YOU'RE NOT BROKEN – THE SYSTEM IS

This is your wake-up call...

The exhaustion.

The irregular and painful menstrual cycles.

The anxious thoughts.

The gut issues.

The overwhelm.

These are not personal failings – they're intelligent responses to a world that's never been designed with women's well-being in mind.

In this section, you'll begin to see with new eyes.

You'll trace the roots of a system that's shaped the way women are taught to relate to their bodies, their emotions, and their worth.

You'll realize that the qualities you've been shamed for – the things that make you 'too much' – are in fact your deepest sources of wisdom.

This is where you stop asking, *What's wrong with me?* and start wondering, *What if nothing's ever been wrong with me?*

This is where you stop pathologizing your body and start listening to it. Questioning the conditioning, decoding your symptoms, and remembering that a woman's sensitivity is not a weakness – it's her superpower.

Chapter 1
REDISCOVERING LOST WISDOM

'The feminine is not a force to be tamed. It is to be honored.'

CLARISSA PINKOLA ESTÉS

'The Natural Superiority of Women' – this was the eye-catching title of a groundbreaking article that appeared in a 1952 edition of the US magazine *The Saturday Evening Post* and was later expanded into a bestselling book. In it, the author, British–American anthropologist Ashley Montagu, boldly declared: 'My many years of work and research as a biological and social anthropologist have made it abundantly clear to me that, from an evolutionary and biological standpoint, the female is more advanced and constitutionally more richly endowed than the male.'[1]

Montagu's work was well ahead of its time, blending science and social commentary to challenge outdated ideas and myths about gender and biology. He knew that calling women 'superior' would provoke a backlash from the male-dominated scientific establishment, yet he didn't flinch from doing so.

Montagu wasn't interested in stirring division between the sexes, though. His goal was to illuminate what the evidence showed: that women possess biological advantages – such as a stronger immune system and greater resilience under stress and emotional strain – that have been critical to the survival of humanity. After three decades of research, he stood firmly by his conclusion, saying that others' attempts to explain it away were not valid.

When I first encountered Montagu's work in my undergraduate anthropology lectures, it felt radical. A portrait of my body that stood in stark contrast to everything I'd been conditioned to believe. At that time, I didn't feel proud to be a woman – in fact, I resented it. I thought we'd drawn the short straw: periods, pain, pressure. I envied men for what I saw as their freedom from our messiness and burdens. A part of me believed Montagu, yet I couldn't shake the dissonance: *If women are built for resilience, then why are so many of us struggling?*

The Female Edge

Today, women have reached unprecedented heights in our education, success, and access to information, yet despite this we've hit a physical and emotional breaking point. For example, in both the US[2] and the UK,[3] women are twice as likely as men to experience depression.

We also have higher rates of insomnia,[4] 50 percent higher stress levels,[5] and comprise 80 percent of autoimmune disease diagnoses.[6] Rates of polycystic ovary syndrome (PCOS),[7] endometriosis,[8] and unexplained infertility[9] are skyrocketing. Girls are starting their periods earlier than ever before.[10] And the global fertility rate has declined by 50 percent in the last 70 years.[11] If we're honest with ourselves, most of us just feel like crap.

Although modern science has continued to validate what Montagu saw so clearly – what women's bodies have always known – this hasn't been communicated effectively to the public. Why? Because the problem lies not in our biology but in the systems surrounding it. Systems that were never built to honor us. Systems that pathologize us, medicalize us, dismiss us, and teach us to doubt ourselves.

*Most of us don't realize how powerful and capable
we are, because we've been conditioned not to.*

We've been taught to mistrust our instincts, suppress our inner knowing, and hand over our authority to someone else. So, when we have that gnawing feeling that there's more to us – more *in* us – we second-guess it. We call it delusion. Selfishness. Narcissism. How dare we want more? How ridiculous to believe that we're powerful.

But the feeling doesn't go away. Emerging research in epigenetics (the science of how our environment and lived experiences can influence which parts of our DNA switch on or off) shows that trauma, stress, and survival patterns can leave molecular imprints on DNA that get passed down through generations.[12,13]

This means that your gut instinct or intuition may be *informed*. While science is still evolving in this area, it's possible that what you feel in your bones is a biological echo. A memory that, thanks to our natural resilience and biological advantages, women were once seen as the keepers of healing wisdom – as intuitive, cultural, and spiritual leaders. And that potential within us didn't vanish, it was *suppressed*.

How Women's Power Was Erased from History

A key part of that suppression was the removal of our access to knowledge. For centuries, women were deliberately kept illiterate, denied the right to read, write, or record their own stories. Our wisdom was passed on orally – shared in circles, in kitchens, at births, and by firesides – while men wrote the books, signed the laws, and decided what counted as 'truth.'

Women's absence from much of recorded history was engineered. Because when a woman is illiterate, she can't document her power; she can't pass it on in the ways the world deems credible; and she can't challenge the written narrative. Unless we understand how that erasure happened, we can't truly reclaim what was always ours. Because once we begin to trace the roots of the system that made us forget, we can finally begin to disentangle ourselves from it.

As Gerda Lerner, who created the first graduate program for women's history in the US, so powerfully warned: 'Women, ignorant of their own history [do] not know what women before them had thought and taught. So, generation after generation, they [struggle] for insights others had already had before them, [resulting in] the constant inventing of the wheel.'[14]

And this is the trap we're still caught in. With so much of our past destroyed, or never recorded at all, unearthing the truth will require more than academic research. We must also turn inward. Learn to trust our intuition. Listen to our bodies. Share with and learn from one another. To piece together the wisdom that lives within us and between us.

> ### *Pause for Self-Reflection*
>
> As you read this chapter, I encourage you to get curious. Notice how your body responds and share what resonates with the women in your life.
>
> - *Ask questions about what you've been told were the role, impact, and achievements of women throughout history – especially within your own lineage and culture.*
> - *What stories have you inherited without ever questioning them?*

This distortion of women's history *matters* because it shapes our understanding of ourselves, the capabilities of our biology, and how we participate in the world we've inherited. As we discover more about the role of women in early societies, we're beginning to see more plainly that the objective facts we were taught about ourselves were shaped by whoever was telling the story – and by whoever was left out of it.

Not 'The Way Things Have Always Been'

Most of us grew up being fed a simplified narrative of humanity's history: Men hunted, women gathered; men led, women followed; men were the ones who built civilizations, while women nurtured them from the sidelines. But this story was never true. Patriarchy has only been around for 1 percent of human history.

In 2023, I was amazed to read a *New York Times* report on research conducted by Dr. Cara Wall-Scheffler, an American biological anthropologist, and her students, which found evidence that in the 63 foraging societies they studied, women hunted in 50 of them – and that 87 percent of that hunting was deliberate rather than opportunistic.[15]

The researchers also found that women adjusted their hunting strategies as they aged – changing weapons, targets, and even hunting partners, depending on their life stage, including whether they had children or grandchildren. (I can almost hear Montagu saying, 'I told you so!')

We're also uncovering more evidence that early societies were neither patriarchal nor matriarchal, in the sense of one gender dominating the other. Instead, they appear to have been egalitarian, matrifocal (centered around women – particularly mothers – as the core of family and social life), or partnership-based. Prioritizing mutual dependence, affiliation, and shared responsibility over power dynamics. Resources were collectively managed, and survival depended on cooperation rather than competition.

We All Come from the Goddess

Spiritually, prehistoric cultures were polytheistic, worshipping gods and goddesses that mirrored the natural world and its cycles. Rather than emphasizing dominance or hierarchy, their spiritual lives reflected an interdependence between masculine and feminine forces.

Art from the Upper Paleolithic Period (c.40,000 to 10,000BCE), such as cave paintings and engravings found in France and Spain, offers us clues about just how central femininity was to early spiritual and cultural life. For example, Canadian paleoanthropologist Genevieve von Petzinger has documented V-shaped motifs that many interpret as representations of the vulva or pubic triangle – symbols of fertility, creation, and feminine power.

And in the Neolithic cultures (from 10,000BCE) she studied, the 20th-century anthropologist Marija Gimbutas identified symbols that linked the feminine with nature, the cosmos, and animals, suggesting a worldview in which women were seen as integral to the natural and cosmic order. Serpents were associated with transformation and regeneration, reflecting the cyclical wisdom of the female body, while spirals and geometric patterns symbolized the rhythms of the universe, mirroring menstrual, lunar, and seasonal cycles.

For Gimbutas, these symbolic connections offered evidence that reverence for women 'encompassed all aspects of social life.'[16] She also identified art and artifacts that centered on a Great Goddess, a sacred feminine figure who had a wide range of roles, including creator, nurturer, protector, and destroyer.

In fact, we know that our ancestors had a deep devotion to the Goddess because 90 percent of the Stone Age sculptures discovered worldwide are stylized depictions of females.[17] Among them is the famous Venus of Hohle Fels, an ivory figurine created between 35,000 and 40,000 years ago (I recommend looking her up – she's amazing).

Why does all this matter? Because today, the world's three major religions – Judaism, Christianity, and Islam – are monotheistic and have male figureheads. However, the idea that God is male is a relatively modern one, and it's not only theological – it's political. When women internalize the belief that God is male, it doesn't just influence our spirituality, it infiltrates our sense of self, our perceived self-worth, our relationship with nature, and our role in the world.

If God is male, then of course it's natural that we outsource our healing, healthcare, intuition, education, leadership, and truth to an external authority – usually a male one. But this wasn't always the way. To remember the Goddess is to remember that you're a powerful leader and creator. You were never meant to seek permission to trust yourself.

You Are the Source

The respect shown by our ancient ancestors for women's bodies extended to their reproductive cycles, which were seen as sacred connections to the moon's rhythms – both unfolding over roughly 28 days. In ancient Egypt, for example, in the village now known as Deir el-Medina, men would even take time off work to care for menstruating wives and daughters, a testament to the societal value once placed on women's cyclical nature.[18]

> *In some ancient traditions, a woman's womb was worshipped as a sacred portal between the physical and metaphysical worlds.*

Creation of the Earth itself was often imagined through the metaphor of birth: stars and galaxies emerging from a cosmic womb. The cosmology of the Vedas, the oldest religious texts of Hinduism (c.1500BCE), beautifully embody this perspective, describing the divine feminine as the 'golden womb'[19] from which all of creation was born.

While it's easy to dismiss such stories as just myth or metaphor, they reflect a profound intuitive understanding that modern science is beginning to echo. Research from NASA's James Webb Space Telescope published in 2025[20] showed that most of the galaxies it studied rotate clockwise – an unexpected finding that's led physicists to question whether our universe might in fact be inside a black hole, nested within a larger universe.

This aligns with earlier theories that claim black holes may function as cosmic wombs, birthing new universes within a greater multiverse.[21] One such theory, proposed by physicist Nikodem Popławski, even suggests that our own universe may have *formed* inside a black hole – essentially, birthed through a kind of cosmic birth canal into a whole new reality.[22]

Women Are Nature

This imagery also echoes across human storytelling and symbolism. For example, many of those who have had near-death experiences describe traveling through a tunnel toward a light – a journey that mirrors birth itself. It's as if both science and spirit are pointing us back to the same truth: What unfolds within women is not separate from the universe but a mirror of what's happening on a cosmic scale.

Okay, so that might sound a little 'out there,' but you must admit the patterns are compelling. And maybe there's something in them worth listening to, because sometimes the point isn't whether an idea is provable but whether it helps us remember something we've forgotten. Something our bodies have always known.

And when we recognize this, we no longer see women as simply *part* of nature – we remember that we *are* nature. We're connected to something mysterious, intelligent, and ultimately unquantifiable. Perhaps that's why, for most of human history, women's bodies – and all they carried – weren't just respected, they were worshipped.

From Sacred to Sinful: The Dawn of Patriarchy

So, how did reverence for the feminine turn into repression? The shift from nomadic lifestyles to settled farming communities around 8000BCE marked a profound turning point. Changes in climate, resource scarcity, and the discovery of fertile lands near major rivers drove migration and competition between groups. Male dominance in trade, politics, physical strength, and military expansion was prioritized, and the concept of ownership (of nature, animals, and people) took hold.

Then, around 3000BCE, cultural models began to transform with the migration of monotheistic Semitic tribes from the Middle East and North Africa. These peoples came from harsh desert environments where survival required domination over, rather than harmony with, nature. Their worldviews reflected scarcity, struggle, and control – values that contrasted starkly with the life-affirming, cyclical wisdom of Goddess-worshipping cultures.

Marginalizing the Feminine

As monotheistic belief systems spread, so too did a new spiritual framework that positioned an all-powerful male God at the center of creation. The feminine was largely erased from religious narratives – and when it couldn't be, it was recast as subordinate, impure, and morally suspect.

The ancient Greeks largely laid the groundwork for this shift by blaming women – such as the mythological first woman, Pandora, who opened the box of misery and evil – for humanity's woes, associating their bodies with frailty and sin.

This theme is mirrored in the Judeo-Christian story of Creation in Genesis, the first book of the Bible. In its original, much earlier, form, this narrative featured the Goddess Ninhursag (protector of life and fertility), a sacred tree symbolizing life, and a serpent representing renewal and transformation, and it honored the feminine as a force of creation and wisdom.

However, in the Genesis account (which scholars believe was written between 950 and 500BCE),[23] the goddess is nowhere to be seen. God the Father assumes sole creative power, Eve is cast as the source of sin and humanity's downfall, and the serpent is vilified as an agent of deception. Completing the transformation of women from sacred to sinful and marginalizing the feminine in spiritual narratives.

Women As Keepers of Healing Wisdom

Women have always relied on strong, interdependent bonds, supporting each other through childbirth, work, and the rhythms of daily communal life, and over time, patriarchal systems of control expanded their reach to target these, as well as women's knowledge and influence.

In the late 12th and 13th centuries, the Catholic Church set up the Inquisition, a tribunal that initially targeted heretics – men and women who defied Christian orthodoxy. But as Church and state institutions grew more centralized, and as anxieties about social order intensified, women became increasingly vulnerable.

This shift accelerated in the wake of the bubonic plague, a pandemic that in the 14th century devastated Europe, killing an estimated 25 to 50 million people. Seen as divine punishment for humanity's sins, the plague provoked a desperate search for scapegoats. Suspicions increasingly turned to women – especially those who lived outside the bounds of patriarchal family structures. Older women, widows, midwives, and healers – many of whom were past childbearing age or were exhibiting menopausal symptoms – were among the most frequent victims.[24]

Persecution, Control, and Silencing

Then came the witch hunts – the investigations and persecutions of alleged witches that took place in European countries and their colonies in the Americas between the 14th and 18th centuries. During this time, women were tortured into naming one another as conspirators. Friendships shattered. Communities fractured. Female networks disintegrated under the weight of fear.

Historians estimate that between 80,000 and 100,000 'witches' were executed across Europe – the vast majority of them women. Countless more were imprisoned, silenced, beaten, or broken. These were women who knew too much. Women who healed, who nurtured, who trusted their bodies and their inner knowing. And for that, they were persecuted by systems that couldn't control them.

Witchcraft was never really the crime – being a powerful woman was. And the fear these women experienced didn't die with them. It lives on today in our hesitation to speak up, in the stories we silence, and in the way we dim our light to stay safe.

We no longer burn women at the stake, but we still shame what's intuitive, feminine, and mysterious. We ridicule the woman who talks about energy and the moon, who trusts her body, uses herbs to heal, and dares to challenge the rational, linear logic of patriarchy.

What this targeting of women shows us is that change – and suppression – takes time. It gathered momentum over centuries, slowly eroding our autonomy, trust, and connection. What began as suspicion turned into policy. What started as fear turned into doctrine. But the persecution of women in the witch hunts was also about power and control. And it paved the way for something even more insidious.

As the Italian–American historian Silvia Federici points out in *Caliban and the Witch: Women, the Body and Primitive Accumulation*, the witch hunts served as a tool for transitioning healthcare, especially reproduction, toward patriarchal and capitalist structures.

From Midwives to the Margins

For most of human history, before medicine was institutionalized, women were the ones people turned to. They worked as midwives, herbalists, and wise women who understood how the body, mind, and spirit were connected. From Siberian shamans to Latin American *curanderas*, they carried knowledge that had been passed down for generations.

Childbirth, in particular, has always been a feminine domain. In ancient artifacts from around the world, women are consistently depicted at the center of birth – surrounded by other women. Roman reliefs show midwives kneeling beside laboring mothers, supporting them through one of the most primal and powerful experiences in life.

However, under the pressures of the witch hunts, women were scapegoated for high infant mortality rates – in reality, the result of inadequate resources. Centuries of accumulated female knowledge and practices were systematically erased or criminalized, and Indigenous knowledge systems were dismissed as 'primitive.'

In the US, with the establishment of the American Medical Association in 1847, midwives were systematically discredited and declared unfit to exercise judgment over their own bodies, let alone those of their patients. A few years later, women were barred from medical schools and excluded from professional associations.

By the early 1900s, obstetricians were able to capitalize on the allure of 'painless childbirth' to draw middle- and upper-class women into hospitals and midwifery was outlawed in some US states. Anesthesia and surgical instruments gave obstetricians absolute control, transforming what had long been a women-led event into a physician-dominated procedure.

By 1935, nearly 75 percent of urban births in the USA took place in hospitals.[25] But rather than making birth safer, this early obstetric intervention often made it more dangerous. Maternal and infant mortality rates increased until the introduction of antibiotics and aseptic techniques in the 1930s and 40s.[26]

The consequences of this shift still reverberate today. British researcher Dr. Andrea Nove estimates that expanding midwife-led interventions in 88 low- and middle-income countries could avert 1.3 million maternal and neonatal deaths annually by 2035.[27]

Doulas and midwives of color are especially instrumental – helping women navigate a medical system shaped by longstanding racial biases and disparities. For example, in the UK, Black women are four times more likely to die in pregnancy and childbirth compared to white women.[28]

For our ancestors, childbirth was not only a physical act but a gateway into a new level of consciousness, strength, intuition, and transformation. To sever women from this communal process is not only to strip them of agency and the support of sisterhood but also to sever them from the wisdom and resilience that birth, at its core, represents.

The New Frontier: Reproductive Rights

So, while it's true that women have gained ground in the realms of education, access to careers, and leadership, the most personal, sacred aspect of our existence – our biology – remains the most politicized, regulated, and contested terrain of all.

In 1973, the landmark Roe v. Wade ruling granted federal protection for abortion in the USA. This right was overturned in 2022 by the Supreme Court and what followed was legal and moral freefall: a patchwork of state bans, many with no exceptions for rape or incest. Abortion clinics shut down. Women were forced to travel hundreds of miles to find care across state lines or risk dying in their cars, turned away from emergency rooms until their lives were considered sufficiently endangered.[29] Doctors faced criminal charges for providing abortion care.

By 2024, several US state legislatures had begun pushing bills that would restrict access to emergency contraception and certain forms of birth control, under the demonstrably false claim that they cause abortions.

As of 2025, there remains no federal protection guaranteeing the right to contraception in the USA, making the message unmistakably clear: Your body is not your own. As Margaret Atwood, author of the eerily prophetic *The Handmaid's Tale*, cautioned in a 2017 essay, historically, 'the control of women and babies has been a feature of every repressive regime on the planet.'

And early in 2025, the US government unveiled a package of financial incentives to encourage childbirth in the face of declining birth rates. Framed as a pro-family initiative, it reveals something much deeper: Women's bodies are being folded into state agendas.[30] When fertility becomes a national asset, women are no longer seen as autonomous individuals but as vessels of demographic strategy. Reproductive freedom ceases to be a right and becomes a duty – one that women are expected to fulfill for the good of the nation.

This latest assault – let's be clear – is not about reproductive rights. It's about the site of our deepest power. And while it's tempting to see these issues as political or legal, at their core, they're spiritual. Existential. They strike at the heart of a woman's sovereignty.

Because when a woman can't choose what happens to her own body, she can't fully choose the direction of her own life. This may be the most overt expression of control, but it's far from the only one. It calls us to look deeper, to examine how the systems that are meant to support women's health are often the ones undermining it.

...

In the next chapter, we'll uncover how patriarchal ideologies became embedded in clinical medicine, and why women's pain is so often dismissed, our symptoms misdiagnosed, and our biology misunderstood.

Chapter 2

HOW PATRIARCHY SHAPED MODERN MEDICINE

'The female body is always assumed to be deviant, when in fact, it is simply different.'

CAROLINE CRIADO PEREZ

Western medicine, like every institution, reflects the values and biases of the culture that created it. And while it has undeniably delivered breakthroughs, it still fails to serve women equitably. For example, women are diagnosed later than men for more than 700 conditions[1] and it can take up to a decade to receive a diagnosis for diseases that affect women disproportionately, such as endometriosis or autoimmune disorders.

These diagnosis and treatment delays are even more pronounced for Black women. Endometriosis, for instance, wasn't even considered a possibility in Black women until the 1970s – decades after it was recognized in white women – due to a toxic mix of systemic racism and enduring myths, including the dehumanizing belief that Black women feel less pain.

In the UK, a 2024 parliamentary inquiry confirmed what many women already know: When presenting with the same symptoms as men, women are twice as likely to be told that it's 'all in their head' or 'just stress,' without further investigation.[2]

So, why do so many women leave medical appointments feeling unseen, dismissed, or disbelieved? Because modern healthcare was built atop the belief that the female body is irregular, overly complex, emotionally unstable, and fundamentally flawed. And those assumptions didn't just shape clinical opinions – they became institutionalized into the foundations of how women are studied, treated, and understood.

Men as the Human Standard

This erroneous belief originated in the 4th century BCE when the ancient Greek philosopher Aristotle claimed that the male body was the human standard and the female body was simply a 'mutilated'[3] version of it (how lovely). He even described women's reproductive anatomy as an inverted version of men's – ovaries were thought to be internal testicles and weren't given their own name until the 17th century.

However, we now know that every human starts with the same basic blueprint in the womb, and it looks more female than male. It's only later, when hormones surge, that a developing body may begin to shift toward the male form. In other words, the original form is feminine. And yet, Western medicine continues to be slow to investigate women's distinct biology, dismissing our cyclical hormones and fluctuating metabolisms as too unpredictable to study.

As a result, medical research has historically prioritized male physiology, while overlooking critical differences between the sexes. Although there's been progress, in many medical schools physiology teaching still focuses on a 'textbook person' – a 21–25-year-old male weighing 154 lb (70 kg) – and offers limited education on the ways biological differences impact health and disease.

One Size Doesn't Fit All

But as it turns out, biological sex influences everything, from the way our immune systems function to how we metabolize medications. For example, hormonal shifts throughout the menstrual cycle can affect how women respond to antidepressants, antibiotics, chemotherapy,[4] and even heart medications – sometimes making doses too strong or too weak.[5]

We've also learned that men's genes tend to change earlier (and more dramatically) with the aging process, while women's genes are often influenced by hormones such as estrogen, especially during their reproductive years.[6] These differences affect the way diseases such as Alzheimer's develop and how our bodies respond to stress and inflammation.[7,8]

Western medicine's one-size-fits-all approach also extends to mental health and trauma. Historically, researchers have generalized men's responses and overlooked the way women experience and process these events. For example, we now know that women are twice as likely as men to develop phobias.[9]

Mind the Gap

Despite humankind's incredible progress in science and technology, research into women's health still lags behind. For example, in the US, the National Institute of Health didn't require women to be included in clinical trials until 1993, and studies involving female animals weren't mandated until 2016 – even for diseases that affect women more often than men. For example, women are 70 percent more likely to experience depression, yet before 2010, studies on brain disorders were five times more likely to use male animals.[10]

Systemic barriers also slow progress. Translating studies into mainstream medical practice can take up to a decade, leaving discoveries gathering dust while women wait for better treatment options.

During my time as a strategy consultant for one of the world's largest academic publishing firms – where I had access to the latest scientific research and leading researchers – I was struck by the stark gender imbalance within the scientific community. Women make up 90 percent of patient-facing healthcare workers around the world[11] yet they account for only one third of researchers[12] and are far less likely to get published or credited in high-impact journals.[13]

This gender bias shapes what gets studied, funded, and ultimately applied in clinical practice, perpetuating significant gaps in our understanding of the female brain and body. This helps explain why progress on researching conditions such as endometriosis and PCOS, and the hormonal transition of menopause, remains so painfully slow.

And why it wasn't until 2023 that the first known study testing the absorbency of menstrual products using blood instead of saline was conducted. It turns out the absorbency of pads, tampons, and other products is significantly different from what labels suggest.[14]

There are still more studies on male baldness than on endometriosis, which is estimated to affect 200 million women globally. One group of researchers even decided to use precious resources to examine physical attractiveness in women with and without the condition. Here's a passage from their study's conclusion that made me both laugh and cry: 'Women with rectovaginal endometriosis were judged to be more attractive... they had a leaner silhouette, larger breasts, and an earlier coitarche (age at first intercourse).'[15]

Our Health Is Relational

It's not my intention to diminish the lifesaving power of Western medicine – as a woman with a life-threatening food allergy, I wouldn't be here without it. However, it does have its blind spots. For example, the more specialized a doctor becomes, the more focused they are on one specific part of the body, and often, the less able they are to see the whole person.

For example, breast cancer patients often report that little attention is paid to their lives beyond their diagnosis, as if the emotional, social, and environmental context of their health is somehow irrelevant.[16] This approach reflects a larger issue: Modern medicine still struggles to treat health as 'relational' – meaning, it often fails to recognize that both illness and healing don't happen in a vacuum.

> *Our health isn't just a set of isolated symptoms or malfunctioning parts; it's shaped by our relationships, environments, histories, and emotions.*

The body is in constant dialogue with everything around it – such as stress, support, nourishment, touch, community, and trauma. When medicine separates the disease from the person's lived experience, it misses a crucial piece of the puzzle: We heal in context, not in isolation.

This disconnect shows up as a tendency to treat symptoms without addressing the full spectrum of what a patient is living through – and what their body may be trying to communicate. Instead of asking *why* we're unwell, and digging for the root, the system is designed to restore our function so we can keep contributing to our workplaces, families, and economies. But this hasn't always been the way it operated.

The Forgotten Prescription

In the 19th and early 20th centuries, Western doctors often prescribed extended rest in the mountains or by the sea to treat ailments like melancholy, nervous exhaustion, or chronic fatigue – recognizing the body's need for nature, beauty, stillness, and space to recover.

Somewhere along the way, that wisdom was replaced by efficiency. Rest was replaced by resilience. Today, we're taught to push through, medicate the pain, caffeinate, and keep performing. Healing has become a race against time, and profit margins. But healing isn't efficient. It asks for slowness, presence, and relief from the very systems that often made us sick in the first place.

In many Eastern traditions, this understanding has persisted. In Japan, for instance, doctors prescribe *shinrin-yoku* (literally, forest bath) – immersing yourself in the atmosphere of a forest – as a therapeutic intervention, demonstrating their understanding that true healing often requires stepping away from the relentless pace of modern life and finding solace in the natural world.

The Myth of Genetic Destiny

During my own navigation of the Western healthcare system, I was told on more than one occasion that my irregular, painful, and heavy periods were 'just genetic.' But this kind of thinking dangerously oversimplifies biology. Here's why.

Genes aren't destiny – they're raw material, like letters on a page. But letters alone don't tell a story. It's the space between them, the context, the *energy*, that gives meaning. And yet, in the patriarchal imagination, genes have become the perfect metaphor: ordered, measurable, linear, fixed. Something to decode, dominate, and ultimately control.

Genetics offered us the illusion of certainty – a tidy explanation that erased the need to ask messier questions about trauma, environment, inequality, poor food quality, or emotional pain (factors we'll explore in Part II of this book). It became a culturally sanctioned way to bypass complexity of the kind that women intuitively understand because we live it every day in our cyclical and emotional bodies.

But real life doesn't operate like a machine or a code. It's dynamic. Fluid. Interdependent. And this is where the emerging science of epigenetics breaks the old notions about genetics wide open. Epigenetics tells us genes don't act in isolation – they respond to the world around them. They're turned on or off by how safe we feel, how nourished we are, how supported we feel in our relationships, how much rest we get, how much stress we carry. In fact, up to 90 percent of disease is driven by these environmental and emotional conditions – not by genetic predisposition.[17] Our biology is responsive, intelligent, and *relational*.

The Missing Piece of the Medical Puzzle

If our genes are responsive, then so too are the systems in the body they inform. One striking example of this came from researchers in Pittsburgh in the US who compared the psychological profiles of women with regular periods and those who had functional hypothalamic amenorrhea (FHA) – a diagnosis for chronically missed periods.

They found that women with FHA reported heightened concerns about dieting, an intense fear of weight gain, and a greater tendency to engage in binge eating.[18] This clearly demonstrates that cultural beliefs, beauty standards, and societal pressures around thinness can shape not only our behavior but also our physiology.

Yet we're conditioned to believe that if we're exhausted, anxious, burned out, or unwell, it's because our bodies are faulty or we've done something wrong – not tried hard enough, not been disciplined enough, not gotten it 'right.' But when you zoom out, the picture becomes clear: Our bodies are responding intelligently to a system that was not built with us in mind.

And perhaps nowhere is this more visible or more misunderstood than in our reproductive system. As many root-cause focussed practitioners have noted, including the bold and brilliant Dr. Jolene Brighten, author of *Is This Normal?*, a woman's menstrual cycle is one of the most sensitive barometers of her overall health. It responds to everything: stress, sleep, nourishment, trauma, safety, and even the quality of her relationships. Our reproductive health isn't separate from the environments we move through – it's the ultimate reflection of them. A mirror held up to the culture we live in, asking us to take a closer look.

• • •

What we've uncovered in this chapter is just the beginning. If patriarchy shaped the foundations of medicine, it also infiltrated the other systems we interact with daily – from the workplace to the wellness industry, and from the media to motherhood. In the next chapter, we'll explore how these cultural forces continue to reinforce disconnection from the body, keeping women small, silent, and sick.

Chapter 3
IMPOSTER SYNDROME OR IMPOSTER SYSTEMS?

*'When women lose themselves,
the world loses its way.'*

GLENNON DOYLE

Patriarchy is often defined as the systemic domination of men over women. But at its core, it's an expression of wounded masculinity – a warped force that infiltrates institutions, cultures, and individual mindsets, and embodies domination, aggression, and control.

None of us, regardless of gender, are immune to the effects of this distorted energy. We see it in workplace cultures, societal norms, cultural expectations, power dynamics, and personal relationships. It shows up in the devaluation of emotional intelligence, care, intuition, and rest – qualities associated with the feminine – and in the lower social status and financial compensation of professions such as nursing, midwifery, and teaching.

Patriarchy disconnects us from our bodies and instincts, while capitalism – which not only emerged alongside patriarchy but was built from it – industrializes that disconnection, turning it into profit. Where patriarchy says 'control,' capitalism says 'exploit.' Where patriarchy says 'suppress the feminine,' capitalism says 'monetize it.'

Masculine and Feminine: Complementary Energies

To be clear, capitalism, in theory, is a system of exchange – not inherently harmful – but the version we live in today is deeply entangled with patriarchal values. Diane Kulju – a writer documenting her healing journey from career burnout on Substack (@littlemammal), and who left Christian evangelicalism over 15 years ago – likens capitalism to a religion in which money is God and retirement is heaven, saying: 'Capitalism as it's practiced now (the belief system, not markets) has morality, sin, punishment, and salvation. And... this myth tells us a lie: that our suffering now will be rewarded by salvation later.'

Perhaps most dangerously, capitalism teaches us to ignore the voice within. To distrust our intuition, our emotions, our sensations, our cycles. It trains us to override the body in order to serve the system.

In contrast to distorted, wounded masculinity, the 'divine masculine' represents direction, order, and truth – a steady, healthier energy that creates the structure and safety necessary for creation (without oppression). The concepts of the divine masculine and divine feminine – archetypal energies that are said to exist in all things – may seem abstract, or even reminiscent of gender stereotypes. However, they have little to do with biological sex and everything to do with balancing complementary energies within us: the interplay of structure and flow, logic and intuition, action and receptivity.

Picture healthy masculine energy as the sturdy banks of a river – providing direction, structure, and containment. While divine feminine energy is the water itself – fluid, creative, adaptable, and life-giving. Both energies are essential. But when masculine energy dominates, structure becomes rigidity. Logic overrides intuition. Action turns into relentless striving without soul, and control replaces trust. As a result of this imbalance, we disconnect from the wisdom of rest, softness, collaboration, and receptivity – the qualities that nourish, heal, and sustain all of us.

How Patriarchy Perpetuates Itself

Patriarchy isn't just a belief system – it's an operating system that breathes through the institutions that shape our lives. From Big Pharma and Big Agriculture to the insurance industry, the wellness sector, and the commodification of care.

These systems aren't neutral, they're mechanisms of extracting labor, energy, time, land, and ultimately, life force. For example, the World Health Organization attributes nearly one third of global deaths – that's 19 million annually – to toxic industries such as fossil fuels, tobacco, alcohol, and ultra-processed foods.[1] Predictable outcomes of a system in which the health of humans and our planet is secondary to profit.

The Digital Cage

Digital technology is one of patriarchy's most cunning disguises. It promises connection, ease, and empowerment, but delivers imbalance and distraction. It offers intimacy in pixels, while leaving us lonelier, more anxious, and profoundly disconnected from ourselves and each other.

Social media platforms don't just sell us products and entertainment; they sell us identities, programming us to chase external approval and silently eroding our confidence. We become commodities, filtered through algorithms that distort our beauty, fragment our self-worth, and reduce our value to how we look and what we have, not who we are.

The legacy of the witch hunts and the policing of female bonds lives on through digital noise that encourages competition over collaboration and distrust over the solidarity of sisterhood.

The illusion of empowerment offered by technology is bolstered by the glorification of urgency and stress. 'Urgent' emails and breaking news alerts flood our nervous systems with cortisol and adrenaline, hormones that evolved to help us survive life-or-death situations by sharpening our focus, fueling productivity, and delivering a fleeting sense of power and purpose. Stress keeps us feeling needed, important, even invincible, for a while, but the crash always comes. And when it does, we're told to look inward – to fix ourselves, biohack our routines, optimize our mornings – rather than question the culture that's driving us to the edge. Chronic stress becomes chronic self-blame.

The Marginalization of Female Pleasure

Digital technology's rapid expansion has far outpaced both social values and ethical regulation – particularly in the way female bodies are represented and consumed. Nowhere is this more evident than in the sexualization of women across media, and increasingly, AI.

These portrayals don't just distort how others see women, they distort how women experience themselves. Instead of teaching us to feel at home in our own bodies, society and social media teach us to focus on our desirability rather than trusting our instincts about what and whom we desire. We're conditioned to prioritize others' satisfaction while disconnecting from our own.

> *There's an internalized belief that women's bodies are instruments of service rather than vessels of creation worthy of reverence.*

Female pleasure is positioned as optional, even taboo, while male pleasure is seen as inevitable and unquestioned. For instance, a content analysis of the website PornHub's 50 most-viewed videos found that only 18.3 percent of the women in them were depicted reaching orgasm, compared to 78 percent of the men. This disparity reflects a broader trend in real-life sexual relationships, where 44 percent of men orgasm every time they have sex, compared to just 16 percent of women.[2]

And when you really sit with the fact that women's pleasure is routinely ignored, it's hard not to see just how systemic this disconnection is. This imbalance teaches us to override our needs, mute our desires, and perform instead of feel. And over time, it erodes our agency – not only in the bedroom but in every area of life where we're taught to accommodate and shrink rather than express ourselves, ask for our needs to be met, and take up space.

Chemical Chaos

When I was 13, I was a competitive swimmer and spent at least two hours a day in the pool, five or six days a week. What I didn't realize back then was that my body was under immense pressure, not just from the physical training but from the invisible load of chlorine and chemical byproducts I was absorbing through my skin and lungs. The result was debilitating period pain that no one could explain.

While my story is of course quite extreme, it reflects a broader truth: We're all swimming in chemicals every single day. From the personal care aisle to the wellness industry, women are disproportionately marketed to and sold products drenched in endocrine-disrupting chemicals (EDCs) – ingredients that mimic, block, or scramble our hormonal signals and overwhelm our body's natural detoxification processes. This is patriarchy in its most palatable form: perfumed, packaged, and very often, pink.

According to a 2015 survey by the Environmental Working Group (EWG), American women use an average of 12 products a day that contain 168 chemicals[3] – a number that's likely climbed, given that nearly 100,000 new chemicals have flooded into our lives over the past 70 years, 86,000 of which have never received vigorous toxicity testing.[4] Men, on the other hand, use an average of six personal care products that contain 85 different chemicals.[5]

The burden isn't shared equally, either. The EWG's 2025 report found that nearly 80 percent of personal care products marketed to Black women were rated as moderate- to high-hazard – highlighting a deeply racialized aspect of chemical exposure.[6]

From cosmetics and cleaning products to clothing, furniture, and the pesticides in our food, EDCs play a role in 80 percent of our deadliest diseases – such as cancer and heart disease – and can alter biology even at extremely low doses.[7]

The scale of this crisis was brought home to me by a 2023 study by Emory University in the US[8] that found measurable levels of PFAS in the blood of newborn babies shortly after birth. This means that babies had been exposed to synthetic chemicals that disrupt crucial processes, such as the growth of tissues and the functioning of their hormones, before they even entered the world.

These EDCs have also been detected in menstrual blood,[9] semen,[10] breast milk,[11] women's ovarian follicular fluid, the placenta,[12] and human brain tissue (with levels up to three times higher in people with dementia).[13]

The Dangers of Ultra-Processed Foods

Our diets are no better. In the past 75 years, we've shifted to consuming large quantities of ultra-processed foods (UPFs), which are often marketed as low-fat, low-carb, gut friendly, and 'guilt-free' but are anything but healthy. Stripped of nutrients essential for hormonal balance, reproductive health, and energy, these foods are loaded with inflammatory ingredients – preservatives, artificial sweeteners, thickeners, and emulsifiers: chemicals known to disrupt gut health, metabolism, and hormones.

They also increase our exposure to EDCs such as phthalates,[14] which leach from packaging and processing equipment into the food itself. The cumulative effect? Early puberty in girls,[15] endometriosis,[16] PCOS,[17] pre-term birth,[18] and estrogen-driven cancers.[19]

Perhaps most disturbingly, many of the food giants that are responsible for UPFs are owned by the same conglomerates that once ran Big Tobacco. No wonder UPFs are engineered in factories to be hyper-palatable, addictive, and shelf-stable for maximum profit. It's not a food system – it's a chemical cartel.

Although awareness is growing and movements are forming, educating yourself on what you're putting into and onto your body, where it comes from, and how it's affecting you is crucial. Don't blame yourself for what you didn't know – even doctors aren't taught in medical school about the harms posed by EDCs and UPFs to human health – just choose to know better now. When you do, you become far harder to exploit.

When Women Become Agents of Patriarchy

What makes patriarchy so deeply entrenched and resistant to change isn't just the systems that uphold it – it's the way it quietly lodges itself inside us. It feeds us contradictions so subtle and insidious they begin to feel like common sense.

Over time, we learn – often unconsciously – to question our desires, censor our instincts, and doubt our own power. Through workplaces, relationships, religion, education, and media, we're conditioned to self-police.

Below is a checklist of just some of the paradoxical 'rules' that women are conditioned to follow. Tick off those rules that you believe in, subscribe to, and which you feel have shaped you:

- ☐ Have faith in your abilities, but don't be boastful.
- ☐ Believe in yourself, but don't be arrogant.
- ☐ Lead with confidence, but make sure you're humble.
- ☐ Be confident, but not *too* confident.
- ☐ Speak up, but don't be aggressive.
- ☐ Be assertive but stay likable.
- ☐ Be visible, but don't promote yourself.
- ☐ Be intelligent, but don't make others feel inferior.
- ☐ Break barriers, but don't upset the status quo.

- ☐ Be empowered but do so in a system that disempowers you.
- ☐ Dress professionally, but not too conservatively, nor provocatively.
- ☐ Be perceived as feminine, sensual, warm, and approachable, but avoid appearing overtly interested in sex.
- ☐ Take care of yourself but prioritize others first.
- ☐ Be a great mother but work as if you don't have children.
- ☐ Don't eat too little, but don't eat too much.
- ☐ Age gracefully, but don't 'let yourself go.'

This constant inner tug-of-war – where no matter what we do, we're either too much or not enough – places enormous pressure on our nervous system, fueling chronic stress, inflammation, and hormonal chaos. Our bodies are breaking down under the weight of trying to be everything for everyone, all the time – while constantly being told we're still not quite right.

Codes of Discomfort

This is why we must ask: Is it imposter syndrome we're battling here, or imposter *systems*? These invisible forces gaslight us into believing our struggles are personal rather than structural. They convince us to shrink ourselves to fit a mold that wasn't made for us – then sell us self-help solutions to cope with the damage.

> *That critical voice in your head? Often, it's not you – it's the system speaking through you.*

And as much as it pains us to admit it, we often become the enforcers of these unspoken rules. Not because we're inherently 'bitchy' or 'nasty,' but because we've been trained to survive within a system that rewards conformity and punishes deviation.

We judge other women for expressing the very parts of themselves we've been taught to suppress. The bold ones. The sensual ones. The unapologetic ones. Maybe you can't even explain why you don't like her. *She's just a lot. There's something about her.*

These phrases become coded language for the discomfort we feel when another woman mirrors the parts of ourselves that we feel, subconsciously, we must hide. We've internalized the belief that being good means being small, and we pass that belief down like a family heirloom.

Tracing the Roots of Our Disconnection

We're all entangled in a dense network of roots – a gnarled and invasive system we can't see that shapes how we think, act, feel, relate to the world, and view ourselves. We inherit them. And we contort ourselves to survive within them. In fact, we're so used to existing in this system that it's only when we attempt to break free or experience a brief reprieve that we can feel just how tightly we're being restrained.

I first experienced what life could feel like outside of that system when I was 14. For an entire school year, I was one of 250 pupils who lived off-grid in remote mountain cabins, segregated by gender, and without technology. No phones, no makeup, no hot showers – unless you chopped firewood and lit a boiler.

Our days were filled with physical labor (such as wood chopping or clearing debris from fire trails), communal meals, and of course, classes. Unlike a typical school program, being smart, good-looking, or athletic wasn't enough here; to survive, you had to contribute – to the unit you lived within, to the community, and to yourself.

This was Timbertop, the outdoor education program of Geelong Grammar School in Australia. The campus's physical challenges are legendary, but what defines Timbertop for those who attend (King Charles III spent time here before starting university), is the way it strips away everything we've been taught to cling to: comforts, distractions, labels, and hierarchies. It breaks you down into the raw materials of yourself, forcing you to confront the truth of who you are.

For the first time in my life, I felt free, and alive in my body – not because I was now honed with muscle, but because I was living. Looking back, it's clear that a year of drinking mountain water, eating fresh, farm-to-table food, and living in a small community where my contributions mattered, awakened something ancient and resilient in me.

My allergies and digestive issues eased. My anxiety and low moods lifted. Periods were discussed openly without shame, and mine regulated for the first time. The unconditional love of sisterhood, paired with male friendships in which I was respected as an intellectual and physical peer, created a sense of capability that I'll carry with me forever.

The Ache of Awareness

After that experience, as I slowly folded back into the 'real' world, I found the sharp contrast between it and the lifestyle at Timbertop enormously destabilizing. I couldn't articulate it yet, but I sensed that something fundamental about the modern way of living was off-balance and was eroding not just the well-being of individuals but the fabric of our collective health. I tried talking about this feeling with friends and family, but most didn't understand what I was reaching for – this is because the majority of people have been trained *not* to see it.

The fiery American feminist and activist Andrea Dworkin mused on this in her book *Our Blood: Prophecies and Discourses on Sexual Politics*: 'Many women, I think, resist feminism because it is an agony to be fully conscious of the brutal misogyny which permeates culture, society, and all personal relationships.'

And so, it became my journey to trace the roots of that discomfort and disconnection – to feel my way into the tangled web of cultural conditioning, systems, and structures that silently shape where and how high women are allowed to grow. What I came to understand is that these limitations are not natural, inevitable, or fixed. But they won't expand to embrace our power unless we demand they do.

Culture can be likened to the soil in which these roots grow. Rich and pervasive, it shapes everything it touches. Seeping into us through every interaction, shaping ideas about who we should be and how we must live. But just as soil can become depleted or polluted, culture too can become toxic, feeding the roots of our disconnection with false narratives.

In Part III, we'll prune back the invasive roots, nourish the ones that sustain us, and begin to restore the cultural soil. This work is not always easy, but it *is* essential. The reclamation of your full power and potential won't be handed to you. It'll be carved out by the questions you dare to ask, the conditioning, beliefs, and habits you choose to unlearn, and the courage you find to trust yourself.

...

In the next chapter, we'll explore the idea of women as an indicator species: biologically sensitive, emotionally attuned, and uniquely equipped to reflect the health of the systems in which we live. Because the feminine doesn't break – it speaks. And it's time we start listening.

Chapter 4
WOMEN AS AN INDICATOR SPECIES

'If you want to know how healthy a society is, look at the well-being of its women.'

GLORIA STEINEM

In my final years at boarding school, as I navigated the pressure of looming exams and the turbulence of puberty, I experienced tidal waves of anxiety. I'd retreat under my duvet for hours, frozen, silently willing the feelings to ease. One day, after I burst into tears during class, a teacher pulled me to one side. At first, he offered a few kind words, but when my emotions didn't quickly tidy themselves away, his tone hardened. He told me I was being hysterical. It landed like a slap – sharp, dismissive, and humiliating. I was drowning, but instead of being met with understanding, I received a centuries-old judgment wrapped in a single word.

The word 'hysteria,' rooted in the Greek word *hystera* (uterus), first appeared in medical texts around 1900BCE. It was formalized by the ancient Greek physician Hippocrates in the 5th century BCE as a diagnosis for unexplained physical and emotional symptoms in women (which he attributed to a 'wandering womb'). The term has endured as a tool to control and diminish women, evolving with the times but never losing its undertone of dismissal.

By the 19th century, hysteria had become a blanket term or diagnosis used to trivialize women's pain and justify their exclusion from public life. Women were too emotional and therefore too irrational and unstable to be trusted with responsibility, autonomy, or credibility. But as it turns out, the profound connection between a woman's emotions and her reproductive health is one of her greatest superpowers.

Signals, Not Symptoms

A 2022 South African study of 237 psychiatrically healthy women aged 18 to 79 found that childhood maltreatment – particularly emotional abuse – was associated with the development of polycystic ovary syndrome (PCOS).[1]

Similarly, a 2018 US study of 60,595 premenopausal women revealed a 79 percent higher risk of developing endometriosis among those who experienced severe physical and sexual abuse during childhood.[2] We also know that menstruating females with higher levels of psychological distress (PD) in adolescence face an increased risk of painful or heavy periods that persist into adulthood.[3]

When you look closely at this research, a remarkable picture emerges – one where women's bodies are reflections of their emotional and psychological states or experiences. Our bodies aren't wired to tolerate systems built on domination, disconnection, profit over well-being, efficiency over sustainability, and toxic expressions of masculinity. They sound the alarm – demanding realignment and pushing humanity to recalibrate to a place of cooperation, respect for the natural world, and matriarchy. Not in the sense of women ruling over men, but in the return to balance and collaboration. Of softness not as weakness, but as strategy.

> *The same traits that make women sensitive to stress also make us powerful agents of change.*

Women are not less capable than men of handling stress; in fact, the evidence often suggests they navigate it more strategically. In the UK, an analysis of

2,800 investors, both male and female, over the course of three years, found that women outperformed men by 1.8 percent annually. Across 20 years, the size of the women's investment pots became a whopping 40 percent greater than that of their male counterparts.[4]

Researchers credited this success to women's long-term perspective, risk-awareness, and ability to avoid impulsive investment decisions driven by emotions such as fear, FOMO, overconfidence, short-term gains, or ego. Unsurprisingly, after the 2008 financial crisis, banks with higher proportions of women in leadership roles, along with countries where female representation in financial governance was greater, endured fewer losses and demonstrated stronger recoveries.[5]

The Power That Shapes Empires

This wisdom isn't new. Genghis Khan, founder of the Mongol empire, which at its peak in the late 13th century was the largest contiguous empire in history, tactically used what historian Jack Weatherford calls 'Daughter Diplomacy'[6] by marrying his three daughters to the kings of newly conquered states. While the men were sent off to battle or distracted with other tasks, the women ruled with skill, stability, and vision.

Even after Khan's death, it was his daughters and granddaughters who preserved the empire's unity by leading armies and reinstating central authority, showcasing the power of the feminine in times of fragmentation. To put this into perspective, the average lifespan of empires led by men over the last 3,000 years has been about 250 years, a milestone the United States approaches in 2025.[7]

We see echoes of this pattern throughout history. In 1789, during the height of the French Revolution, it was the mothers, wives, and market women of Paris who marched on Versailles – demanding bread, justice, and dignity for their starving families. They didn't just ignite a pivotal moment in the Revolution; they reminded the world that when women rise in defense of life, empires tremble.

And modern research continues to reflect this truth. Studies show that when women are in leadership or decision-making roles, outcomes improve – whether in politics, business, or community health. So, if history teaches us anything, it's that when the feminine is honored, stability strengthens. And when it's dismissed or suppressed, systems inevitably unravel.

Women's Biological Brilliance

Women don't just absorb stress – we adjust, adapt, and find new ways to survive. And while those adaptations can come with a price, they're evidence of a remarkable biological intelligence. A great example of this type of adaptation is a phenomenon called hypermutation, which has been observed in bacteria under extreme stress.[8] When threatened by antibiotics, the bacteria don't just give up and collapse, they accelerate their mutation rate, increasing the likelihood of developing antibiotic resistance.

This is the biological drive to survive at all costs, a principle that also plays out in women's bodies. As the Canadian–American physician Dr. Sharon Moalem suggests in his book *Survival of the Sickest*,[9] many of the conditions that seem harmful to us today may have originally evolved as protective adaptations forged in times of famine, environmental hardship, or emotional strain.

The Drive to Survive

When we apply this lens to women's health, it reveals that some of the challenges we're facing now are not dysfunctions but expressions of deep biological intelligence:

- Heightened immune responses in women may once have protected against infections during pregnancy or childbirth, but today these overactive immune systems are implicated in autoimmune conditions,[10,11] and as we've recently discovered, endometriosis, which is now being understood as both an inflammatory and immune-related disorder.[12]

- Longer menstrual cycles or the loss of a cycle (as seen in PCOS) might have conserved energy during times of famine or stress, delaying reproduction until conditions were safer.

- Women with PCOS often have higher testosterone levels, greater muscle mass, and enhanced stamina – traits that would've been advantageous in harsh, physically demanding environments. In fact, a disproportionately high number of elite female athletes, including Olympic medalists, have PCOS.[13]

What we're seeing is that the traits which were once advantageous for survival are now colliding with modern-day stressors: chronic overwhelm, ultra-processed diets, environmental toxins, and the relentless pressure to perform. Our brilliant evolutionary tactics, once lifesaving, have become sources of suffering in a world that no longer supports our biology.

We Aren't Defective, We're Responsive

Clearly, women's bodies aren't broken. Instead, they're responding with precision to an environment that is. In ecology, an indicator species is an organism – bacteria, plant, or animal – whose presence, absence, or health reflects the condition of the environment around it. These indicator species are sensitive to disruption, and their decline is often the first warning sign that something in the ecosystem is off. Frogs, for example, are considered an indicator species because their porous skin and complex life cycles make them highly responsive to environmental toxins and shifts.

Women are the indicator species of our human ecosystem. We're responsive. But the longer we remain in survival mode, the more deeply it embeds itself into our biology and alters brain function[14] – suppressing activity in the hippocampus (the brain's center for memory and learning) while hyperactivating the amygdala, which governs fear and threat detection.

Over time, this rewires the brain so that the stress response is activated even when no threat is present. Essentially, stress becomes a way of being – showing up as hypervigilance, overachievement, or emotional reactivity. As one of my clients, Emily, remarked: 'Hypervigilance is my entire personality. I don't know any other way of existing.' And when you think about it, isn't hypervigilance one of the most effective ways to keep women disconnected from their full power and potential? By trapping them in a permanent state of survival.

Our Bodies Are Barometers of Balance

Why does women's reproductive health suffer in particular? We'll dive deeper into this in the next chapter, but first, it's important to understand that reproduction demands immense energy over nine months of gestation, sometimes putting a woman's survival at risk. So, when the body senses any threat – whether physical, emotional, or relational – it conserves energy for more essential functions. Ovulation pauses. Menstrual cycles become disrupted. Fertility drops. Pregnancy may even terminate. The body, in its wisdom, does what it must to protect us.

Ancient cultures understood intuitively that women's bodies are barometers of balance. Our ability to menstruate, conceive, and carry life was seen as an indicator of whether a society was in harmony or out of sync. In ancient Greece, land fertility and female fertility were intertwined. If women or the land stopped flourishing, rituals were performed to restore balance, often honoring goddesses like Demeter. In Native American traditions, a woman's fertility is a spiritual and ecological signal – reflecting the well-being of the whole tribe.

So, when we ask ourselves what our suffering is trying to tell us, the answer has always been there. But patriarchy – and its offsprings capitalism and colonization – don't want us to hear it. They gaslight us, distract us, and sell us solutions to problems that they created, all while keeping us small and sick enough not to probe too deeply.

But now we see clearly that our breaking point is a biological protest against a way of living that's fundamentally incompatible with life. We must heed the wisdom of American astrophysicist Neil deGrasse Tyson, who said: 'We are all connected; to each other, biologically. To the Earth, chemically. To the rest of the universe, atomically.'[15]

...

To better understand these signals that our bodies are sending, we need to decode the language our bodies speak. The next chapter provides a missing biology lesson, revealing how our hormones translate the pressures we've been carrying.

Chapter 5
THE BIOLOGY LESSON THAT WOMEN DESERVE

'The most common way people give up their power is by thinking they don't have any.'

ALICE WALKER

During their lifetime, 80 percent of women will experience a hormone imbalance.[1] That number is too big to dismiss as 'just part of being a woman.' Something deeper is going on – not just in our bodies but in the way that society shows us to respond to them.

Instead of being taught to understand the underlying causes of our hormonal symptoms, we're handed quick fixes: birth control, supplements, adaptogens, tonics. A billion-dollar wellness industry has been built around the idea that our bodies need to be managed or corrected – selling us Band-Aids for issues that are deeply rooted in the way we're expected to live, work, and perform.

We're told to biohack our way out of burnout, to green-juice away our discomfort, to optimize ourselves into balance, all without ever asking: *Why are so many women's bodies speaking this loudly in the first place?* This obsession with individual solutions keeps us disconnected from ourselves, from each other, and from the deeper *why* behind the symptoms we carry.

Hormones: Our Body's Messengers

Take hormonal birth control. A 2022 review estimated that 151 million women of reproductive age were using oral contraceptives, many of them to manage symptoms such as pain or heavy bleeding.[2] I was on the pill for over a decade before I had the knowledge, support, and stability to stop it and begin navigating my symptoms and restoring my natural cycle.

Let me be clear – hormonal contraception has been a powerful tool in granting women freedom, choice, and control over our futures, and I fully support every woman's right to choose what's best for her. But too often, it's prescribed not as empowerment but as erasure. Period pain? Acne? Irregular cycles or PCOS? Mood swings? Try the pill. There's rarely any investigation into why these symptoms occur in the first place.

There's not enough education about key consequences such as nutritional depletion.[3] And when the side effects arrive – anxiety, depression, loss of libido, emotional numbness – we're told it's worth it. That it's better than the alternative. But the alternative we're comparing it to is a misunderstood, misrepresented, and mistreated version of our biology.

Your menstrual cycle is a medically recognized reflection of your overall health – a feedback system, a monthly report card. When you suppress it, you don't just turn off ovulation, you silence the body's communication network. So, in this chapter, you're going to reclaim your biological literacy. Learning what you were never taught: that your hormones are not the problem.

Hormones are the body's master messengers, impacting everything – our energy, digestion, metabolism, immune system, and ability to sleep. Most importantly, they interpret stress, translating what's happening in our environment, relationships, and inner world into physical feedback. In other words, hormones tell you how your body's responding to the world around you.

The Hormone Hierarchy

We're not only going to talk about what hormones do, but about what they *reveal*. They show us where our lives are out of balance, where stress is building up, and where our needs have been neglected for too long. So, if your symptoms have never quite made sense, or if you've felt as if you're not operating at full capacity, this is your chance to finally understand what your body is trying to say.

Your body relies on more than 50 different hormones working together all the time, but not all hormones have the same level of influence. Let's break this down.

Tier 1 Hormones: The Foundational Regulators

Some hormones react to changes happening in your body, while others are more foundational, setting the stage for how your entire hormone system functions. When these foundational hormones – cortisol, insulin, oxytocin, and dopamine (what I call the Tier 1 hormones) are out of balance, everything else can start to fall apart.

Cortisol – The Stress Hormone

Cortisol is the most influential hormone in the hierarchy. Produced by your adrenal glands, it's your body's built-in alarm system – keeping you alive by responding to stress. When your body senses danger, cortisol kicks in, flooding your system with energy to survive the threat. It shifts your body into high-alert, prioritizing survival over non-essential processes such as digestion, reproduction, healing and self-repair.

Insulin – The Energy Storage Hormone

Insulin helps control your blood sugar levels and how your body stores energy from the food you consume. When it's out of balance, it can lead to issues such as metabolic challenges, inflammation, weight gain, painful periods, and conditions like PCOS.

Oxytocin – The Safety and Connection Hormone

Released through touch, intimacy, and bonding, oxytocin calms the stress response by reducing cortisol levels. This promotes healing and enhances trust and empathy. New research also shows that oxytocin can influence moral emotions and decision-making by increasing feelings of fairness. This makes us more inclined to act in ways that support social harmony – revealing how deeply our hormonal health is tied to both emotional well-being and our ability to make decisions that align with our values.[4]

Dopamine – The Motivation and Reward Hormone

Dopamine drives focus, energy, and your ability to follow through on habits that serve you. Low dopamine is linked to procrastination, emotional reactivity, impulsivity, and disconnection from a sense of purpose. Artificial stimulation from social media, shopping, and sugar hijacks this system, making it harder to maintain hormone-supportive routines such as healthy eating, proper sleep, and regular exercise.

Tier 2 Hormones: The Builders

DHEA and pregnenolone, hormones produced by the adrenal glands, act as precursors – the raw materials that the body uses to produce other essential hormones, including estrogen, progesterone, and testosterone. Their balance is highly influenced by the health and balance of Tier 1 hormones, especially cortisol and insulin.

Tier 3 Hormones: The Specialists

Estrogen, progesterone, testosterone, thyroid hormones, and melatonin are often the most tested and treated hormones, but they're also the most easily thrown off course. These specialist hormones sit at the top of the hormone hierarchy, and their balance depends heavily on the stability of the foundational Tier 1 and builder Tier 2 hormones.

Disruption of Tier 3 Hormones

When those Tier 1 and 2 hormones are imbalanced, the Tier 3 hormones are the first to create symptoms – whether it's irregular cycles, mood swings, weight gain, low libido, insomnia, or fatigue. Here are two examples of how this works in practice:

Cortisol and progesterone (a key hormone for cycle regulation, sleep, and calm): These are made from the same building hormone, pregnenolone. When you experience high levels of stress, your body prioritizes cortisol production to keep you safe. This means there are fewer resources available to make progesterone. The result can be irregular or missing cycles, PMS, anxiety, insomnia, and fertility challenges.

Insulin and estrogen: Estrogen helps your body use insulin effectively and keep blood sugar balanced. But when estrogen levels drop – during times of stress or in perimenopause – your body becomes more insulin resistant. That makes it harder to manage energy, weight, and inflammation.

On the flip side, chronically elevated insulin (from poor diet, binge-restrict cycles, or chronic stress) can raise circulating estrogen levels and reduce the proteins that regulate it. This disrupts your cycle and increases the risk of estrogen-dominant conditions such as heavy periods, fibroids, and PMS.

What Are Your Hormones Telling You?

When it comes to hormones, we tend to think only in biological terms – test results, symptoms, diagnoses. But hormonal imbalances often begin upstream, in the psychological and social realms. Patterns like perfectionism, toxic relationships, and systemic inequality don't just shape how you feel – they shape your internal chemistry.

Disruption of Tier 1 Hormones

At the same time, when your hormones are disrupted, it becomes harder to regulate your emotions, trust yourself, or show up in your relationships, which can then reinforce the patterns that contributed to the imbalance in the first place.

Biological, psychological, and social factors are deeply interwoven and bidirectional. That means your symptoms can't be understood in isolation – they're part of an intelligent, adaptive system. Below, I've explained how disruption of the four Tier 1 hormones reflects this interconnected reality. Use these signs to help you start to decode the deeper messages your body is sending you.

Cortisol

Biological: inflammation, sleep deprivation, nutrient deficiencies, gut imbalances, thyroid disorders, autoimmune conditions, and insufficient micronutrients (like magnesium, B vitamins, and omega-3s).

Psychological: trauma, anxiety, perfectionism, people-pleasing, hypervigilance, internalized guilt for prioritizing self-care, emotional labor in relationships (the invisible effort of managing others' emotions, needs, and comfort).

Social: gender pay gaps, caregiving responsibilities, toxic relationships, insufficient maternity leave or support, cultural expectations as caregivers, sexual harassment, and racial or gender discrimination.

Insulin

Biological: blood sugar imbalances, PCOS, inflammation, and sedentary lifestyles.

Psychological: emotional eating, body shame, and trauma around food.

Social: diet culture, food insecurity, and societal glorification of hustle culture.

Dopamine

Biological: nutrient deficiencies (such as iron, B6, and folate), poor sleep, hormonal imbalances, undiagnosed ADHD.

Psychological: Perfectionism, burnout, low self-worth.

Social: glamorized overachievement, digital overload, lack of meaningful creative outlets.

Oxytocin

Biological: stress, trauma, lack of intimacy, lack of orgasms, and hormonal imbalances.

Psychological: fear of rejection, loneliness, or struggling to trust others.

Social: limited postpartum care, digital connection, and social expectations of sacrifice.

While this list of disruptors isn't exhaustive, it's been intentionally curated to spotlight the forces that uniquely and disproportionately affect women. Now, please don't let it overwhelm you – the point isn't to add more to your plate but to help you see just how deeply your health is impacted by the systems in which you live.

> *Pause for Self-Reflection*
>
> Before you move on, take a moment to sit with the list of hormone disrupters above and then respond to these questions in your journal:
>
> - *Which patterns feel familiar in your own life?*
> - *Where might your body be asking for more support?*
> - *Are there any disruptors that surprised you?*

In Part III, I will walk you through how to begin untangling these forces, step by step.

A Note on Hormone Testing

If you're curious about your hormone levels, please keep in mind that while functional lab work can provide valuable insights, bloodwork often doesn't show dysfunction until it's pretty advanced. Why? Because the body is incredible at keeping blood volume stable, even when there's dysfunction happening.

So, you don't want to wait until bloodwork shows something's wrong before acting. If your results come back 'normal' but you still don't feel right, trust your instincts. Use functional lab work as a guide, not as a definitive answer. It's simply feedback on where you are right now. Learn to listen to your body – don't wait for lab results to confirm what you already know.

• • •

Now that you understand how the foundational hormones cortisol, insulin, dopamine, and oxytocin set the stage for your overall health, in the next chapter we'll shift our focus to specialist, reproductive hormones. We'll also look at why aligning with our natural rhythms is essential for lasting well-being.

Chapter 6
A 'SUPERIOR' BIOLOGICAL BLUEPRINT

'Everything in nature is a cycle.
Why should women be any different?'
MIRANDA GRAY

Another pivotal moment in my healing journey came about through a woman I deeply admired – Sylvia, a senior executive I met while working at a CEO advisory firm. Brilliantly capable, she led an all-male team and had achieved the kind of corporate success I thought I wanted for myself at the time. But beneath her sharp, glamorous, and composed exterior was a woman quietly battling burnout, loneliness, and the weight of a dream she was running out of time to fulfil.

In her early 40s and single, and after years of pouring herself into work, Sylvia decided to pursue motherhood on her own. She found a sperm donor, started IVF, and after multiple failed attempts, she finally conceived. Her joy was unmistakable, and she shared the news with us earlier than she probably should have.

However, despite hailing her pregnancy as a 'miracle,' Sylvia didn't carve out space to let her body soften into the shift. Instead, she stuck to the rhythm of spreadsheets and strategy meetings, juggling work, hormones, and hope. Her mother moved in to support her, but still, she pushed forward, trying to do it all. And then, she lost the baby.

Sylvia was convinced that her pregnancy terminated because she didn't slow down; only in the wake of that loss did she take extended leave. And that, I believe, is the part we don't talk about enough. When a woman is struggling to conceive, the first piece of advice she usually hears is 'just go on holiday.' Because, whether we admit it or not, we know that the female body cannot create new life when it's contorting to fit systems that ignore its needs.

Our Cyclical Rhythms

But it shouldn't take stepping away from your career to access your fertility. Our ancestors worked; they moved their bodies, tended the land, and raised children under extremely harsh conditions. But they also lived in rhythm with nature, in a community, and in cycles that honored the seasons. The problem is our environment, which ignores the inherent needs of female biology and penalizes the very rhythms that make us powerful.

Of all the ways our society's systems disrupt women's hormones, one of the most overlooked – and urgent – is that we are cyclical beings, forever changing and adapting, and yet we're expected to live as if we're linear and predictable.

Nearly two years after my reckoning at the World Economic Forum, hearing Sylvia's story gave me the courage I needed to finally step away from the world of consulting to fully focus on healing my Polycystic Ovary Syndrome (PCOS) – and begin living in alignment with my body's true biological rhythm. That decision marked the beginning of a profound shift. As I began to sync with my own hormonal rhythm, I realized how deeply our cultural norms are modeled on a male biological template.

To understand why this matters, let's look at the key differences between male and female hormonal cycles, both daily and monthly, and how they shape everything from energy and focus to stress, creativity, and rest.

Daily and Monthly Cycles: Men vs. Women

Men's hormonal cycles are primarily driven by a 24-hour internal clock (the circadian rhythm) that regulates physical, mental, and behavioral changes throughout the day. Levels of hormones such as testosterone and cortisol peak early morning to fuel energy, focus, mood, and stress regulation, making men naturally optimized for productivity during the first half of the day.

As the day progresses, these hormone levels gradually taper off, contributing to a natural decline in energy and mental sharpness by evening. Notably, men's brains also experience daily fluctuations, shrinking by about 0.6 percent by the end of the day and resetting overnight.[1] This consistent daily pattern aligns well with a traditional 9-to-5 work schedule (surprise, surprise), which maximizes men's cognitive performance and efficiency.

Women's Hormonal Fluctuations

Women, on the other hand, operate on a dual rhythm during their reproductive years: the circadian rhythm, which regulates daily cycles like wake–sleep patterns, and the infradian rhythm, which governs the menstrual cycle.

Spanning an average of 28 days (though it can vary from 26 to 35 days), the infradian rhythm is anchored by two key events: ovulation (peak fertility) and menstruation/period (release and renewal). As the illustration on the following page shows, throughout the month women's hormones fluctuate dynamically, creating distinct energy, mood, and cognitive shifts across four key phases: menstruation, follicular, ovulation, and luteal (premenstrual).

This means women are hormonally different from week to week, even day to day, with each phase likened to nature's seasons: menstruation/winter; follicular/spring; ovulation/summer; luteal (premenstrual)/autumn.

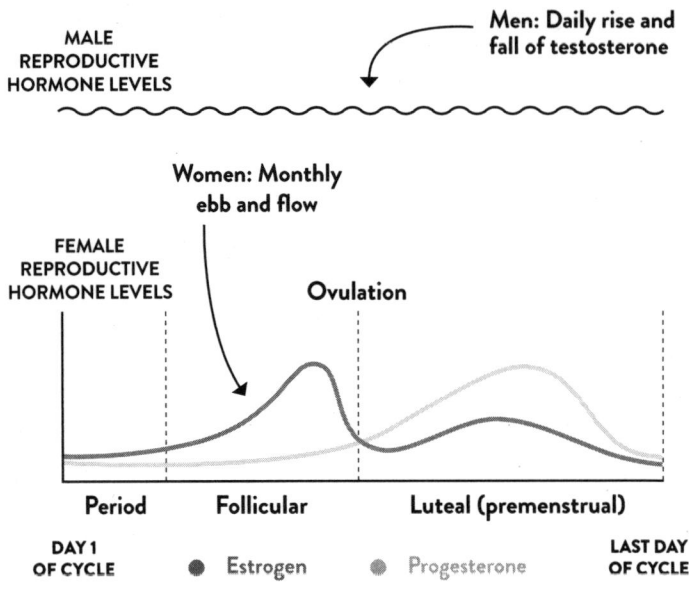

Male vs. female sex hormone cycles

Inbuilt Feminine Resilience

The fluctuations during these four phases are far from minor. One study of 60 women found that brain activity in regions associated with cognition, emotional regulation, and stress response shifts significantly throughout the month, with some experts estimating the brain changes by about 25 percent,[2] allowing women to harness different strengths at different times.

For both men and women, these rhythms provide natural access to masculine and feminine energies. Men's steady hormonal rhythm supports consistent action and focus (masculine), while women's dynamic monthly cycle aligns them with periods of productivity and creation (masculine) as well as reflection and receiving (feminine).

This is where more of women's untapped power lies. Yes, men can learn this reflective capacity, but for us, it's built into our biology. That's why, throughout history, women were respected as pillars of community leadership.

> *Women's cycles are project managers, checking in to tell us when something isn't sustainable – whether it's our diet, environment, pace, or the systems we live within.*

It's no coincidence that men who are married to women,[3] or who have daughters, live longer (one study found a man gained 74 weeks of life per daughter).[4] Women bring a natural understanding of the importance of rest that elevates the well-being of everyone around them. But of course, when our hormones are out of balance, it becomes harder to hear that wisdom.

Your Body, Their Business

For women, understanding these cycles isn't only vital for personal empowerment – it also enables us to recognize how this intimate knowledge is being used against us. While researching for this book, I connected with several successful women in the FemTech industry who warned me that many of the most popular menstrual-tracking apps had sold users' cycle data to marketing firms, often without clear consent or transparency.

For example, a 2019 report by Privacy International[5] uncovered that popular apps like Period Tracker and Flo shared sensitive data with companies such as Facebook and Google, allowing them to target marketing campaigns based on hormonal fluctuations, pregnancy, and sexual activity.

It's disturbing that while most women are never taught the full significance of their cyclical rhythms, capitalistic corporations monetize this biological insight. If we don't reclaim this knowledge for ourselves, we remain vulnerable to manipulation, allowing companies to influence our decisions and behaviors through data they understand better than we do.

Seasonal Cycles

Men, too, suffer under our current linear model by being severed from their own need for rest. Practically every other mammal slows down, conserves energy, or hibernates during the winter months, yet in our infinite wisdom, we humans decided to maintain summer productivity standards year-round.

And when we inevitably struggle to keep up, we label it seasonal affective disorder (SAD) – a form of depression that typically occurs during winter – and treat it as dysfunction rather than honoring it as a signal to pause, restore, and recalibrate.

Women, often more attuned to the natural fluctuations in their mood and energy, are better equipped to recognize and adapt to seasonal shifts, while men often lack the frameworks or support systems to identify and address these changes, leaving them more vulnerable to burnout and emotional distress.

Life Cycles

Men typically experience just two main hormonal transitions throughout their life: puberty and a gradual drop in testosterone as they age (a phase called andropause). Meanwhile, women can experience up to eight – puberty, the reproductive years, pregnancy, postpartum, breastfeeding, perimenopause, menopause, and postmenopause.

Each stage brings shifts in the body and mind, helping women adapt to their changing roles and challenges while connecting them more deeply to their strength and purpose. For example, during pregnancy, the brain undergoes remarkable changes, including a reduction in gray matter in areas linked to social understanding and bonding.[6] While this might sound concerning, it's actually a fine-tuning process that sharpens maternal instincts, empathy, and social awareness, preparing women for caregiving and protection.

But these changes don't stop at nurturing – they also boost emotional intelligence, multitasking, and collaboration.

Women's capacity for physiological renewal also extends to menstrual blood and placental tissue. Once dismissed as shameful, dirty waste, they're now emerging as sources of cellular healing and regenerative medicine (because, of course, women are a source of miracles). Menstrual blood, for instance, contains mesenchymal stem cells (MSCs) with potential for treating strokes and type 1 diabetes.[7,8] Similarly, placental-derived stem cells have shown promise in wound-healing and neurological treatments.[9]

Suddenly, ancient practices don't seem so strange. In Traditional Chinese Medicine, the placenta (*zi he che*) is often consumed to boost energy, support fertility, and restore hormonal balance. Likewise, Ayurveda regards the placenta as a life-giving substance rich in *prana* (vital life force), promoting healing after childbirth.

Menopause

Menopause is a final and profound recalibration. A 'second spring' that frees women from reproductive demands and redirects their energy toward new roles and purposes. In Traditional Chinese Medicine, this term speaks to a woman's return to herself: no longer cycling outward but spiraling inward into wisdom, creative power, and sustained clarity.

Menopause is an evolutionary maturation – a rite of passage that our culture has pathologized, but which nature designed as a gateway to deeper power. One key biological shift is streamlining of the brain, a process that enhances focus, emotional resilience, adaptability, and problem-solving.[10]

These changes align with the 'grandmother hypothesis,' an evolutionary theory which suggests that menopause primes women to step into roles as mentors, nurturers, and system-shapers. This key role may also explain why women outlive men; their extended lifespans provide essential support, from caregiving to the transmission of knowledge, ensuring the survival and success of future generations.

For previous generations, menopause typically marked a time when children had moved out of the home, and many women were embracing the joys of becoming grandmothers. It was a natural transition into a new phase of life, often accompanied by a sense of freedom and space to focus on personal growth and well-being.

Today, the situation is very different. The increased sensitivity to cortisol that accompanies menopause offers women an opportunity to let go of what's no longer serving them, to clear the clutter, and set stronger boundaries. Yet many women are navigating this transition while managing late motherhood, reaching peaks in their careers, or juggling households where their hormonal shifts often coincide with those of their teenage children. What they need is deep support and nourishment, not the added weight of carrying the heaviest possible load. It's no wonder so many women feel overwhelmed and burned out.

Generational Cycles

When women aren't supported in moving through these transitions, we all feel the ripple effects. Through mitochondrial inheritance – the transmission of mitochondrial DNA passed exclusively from mother to child – women carry and transmit the energetic imprint of their lived experience: from stress to nourishment, trauma to joy.

These biological messages shape how future generations adapt to the world they're born into. When a woman lives without safety, under stress, her body cannot fully repair or replenish, and her mitochondria (the energy centers in every cell) carry that depletion forward. But when women are truly supported, with agency and reverence, an inheritance of burnout can become a legacy of vitality. We gift not only ourselves but future generations – a blueprint of resilience in a world that deeply needs it.

•••

In the next chapter, we'll explore what it would look like to create new systems that not only support women's biological design but also challenge the deeply ingrained structures that have limited our potential for far too long. It's time to rethink our pursuit of gender equality, and what it takes to build systems that promote well-being and success for everyone.

Chapter 7
IT'S TIME FOR GENDER EQUITY

'Women must learn to play the game as men do.'
ELEANOR ROOSEVELT

Our world isn't broken, just unfinished – built on a system that honors only half of humanity's story and half of its potential. Under less-than-optimal conditions (to put it kindly), women have adapted and contorted themselves to fit so well that across much of the developed world, young women are even starting to leave men behind.[1] They're excelling in education, earning degrees at higher rates, and increasingly balancing careers with caregiving, all while holding the emotional architecture of their families and communities intact.

This extraordinary feat is the result of a courageous and necessary effort to advance gender justice by focusing on equality, expanding women's access to education and professional opportunities under the assumption that aligning with men in certain domains would help close the gap between genders.

But the scales remain uneven. Men still hold the advantage when it comes to economic power,[2] while women continue to shoulder the bulk of unpaid emotional and domestic labor.[3] And in a phenomenon called the glass cliff, women who have broken through the glass ceiling are often appointed to leadership positions in businesses that are teetering on the edge of failure, only to be blamed when collapse proves inevitable. Meanwhile, men glide upward on the glass escalator, advancing seamlessly, even in fields traditionally dominated by women.[4]

No country in the world has achieved full gender equality, and at the current pace, it could take centuries to close the gap. With 2030 looming as the UN's global benchmark to achieve 'gender equality and empower women and girls,' we're not just falling short, we're actively losing ground in countries as diverse as the USA and Afghanistan.

And while it's tempting to frame gender equality as a political or economic issue, it's also deeply cultural and spiritual. Around the world, gender-based violence remains the ultimate expression of patriarchy's fear of feminine power. Domestic abuse, femicide (the murder of women or girls because of their gender), coercive control, and state-sanctioned oppression are attempts to suppress the brilliance, autonomy, and embodied excellence of women.

From Equality to Equity

It's not just women who are struggling – unfolding in parallel is a growing crisis of disenfranchisement among men. Many, especially those who are falling behind in education or employment, are gravitating toward reactionary ideologies and populist movements that promise restored control and identity in a rapidly changing world.[5,6] This widening gender divide demands deeper questioning: *What kind of progress are we really creating? And who is it serving?*

In 2025, during an appearance on Joe Rogan's podcast, Meta CEO Mark Zuckerberg argued that our society needs more focus on masculine qualities: 'I just think we've kind of swung culturally to that part of the spectrum where it's all like, "Masculinity is toxic. We have to get rid of it completely",' he said, and then added, 'I think having a culture that celebrates the aggression a bit more has its own merits' and 'a lot of men feel neutered and emasculated.'[7]

While Zuckerberg is right to acknowledge the discomfort some men feel in a culture that increasingly questions masculinity, it's clear he's missing the deeper point. In these comments, he's conflating the demonization of *toxic masculinity* with a rejection of masculinity as a whole – suggesting we've gone too far by labeling traits such as aggression as inherently bad.

But this isn't about erasing masculinity – it's about redefining it. What's being called into question isn't strength or ambition but domination, emotional repression, and unchecked power. Of course, acknowledging this would require Zuckerberg to face the fact that his business, and the systems it supports, perpetuate toxic masculinity.

Recognizing Our Differences

As Dr. Robert Augustus, a psychotherapist and author who focuses on integrating masculinity in a healthy, balanced way, teaches, true masculinity isn't about dominance or aggression. It's about strength and depth, standing in integrity, and holding space for others, especially the feminine. It's about being a protector, not a controller.[8]

Likewise, feminine energy isn't weak or passive. It's intuitive, creative, and attuned to meaningful connection – qualities that are not only powerful but essential in leadership, especially for those at the helm of global social networks. If we continue to cling to outdated definitions of masculinity and femininity, we'll keep recreating the same broken systems: toxic workplaces, disconnected people, and a divided culture.

> *Leadership that blends strength with empathy, and action with reflection, isn't just more effective, it's what the world urgently needs.*

Time and experience have taught me that chasing equality without recognizing biological difference doesn't liberate women, it suppresses us. As the poet and activist Audre Lorde says in her book *Sister Outsider*: 'It's not our differences that divide us. It's our inability to recognize, accept, and celebrate those differences.'

True progress will never be made by simply allowing women to fit into the systems that already exist. We need to redesign and expand them entirely – shifting our focus from equality to *equity*. Creating a world where women are honored as the intuitive, cyclical, regenerative leaders they are. But that kind of transformation doesn't begin with governments or institutions. It begins with us – when we stop chasing power outside of ourselves and start reclaiming it from within. And to truly understand the depths of this reclamation, we must confront one of history's most deliberate erasures.

Power Was Never Outside of You

I was raised Catholic – not in an overly strict way, but enough that Church was woven into the rhythm of my early life. But as I dutifully listened to sermons and sang hymns, something didn't sit right. I experienced a subtle discomfort, a sense that something essential was missing.

That eventually grew into disillusionment, and I began to question everything I'd been taught. By my late teens, I'd stepped fully into atheism, convinced that religion had nothing meaningful to offer me. Now I understand what that discomfort really was. It was the absence of Mary Magdalene's voice. The absence of ours.

Christianity, with its 2.3 billion followers, remains one of the most influential institutions, shaping values, identities, and moral frameworks around the world. Yet, as we touched on in Chapter 1, woven into its foundations is a calculated suppression of the feminine, and nowhere is this more evident than in the treatment of Mary.

In the 4th century, an edict was issued to destroy all copies of non-canonical gospels, including the Gospel of Mary (which recounts Jesus's teachings after his resurrection). Why? Because it challenged the male-dominated hierarchy and patriarchal narrative. Mary Magdalene wasn't a repentant prostitute – a story fabricated by Pope Gregory I in 591 CE – but Jesus's closest disciple (controversially, some scholars claim she was his lover or wife),[9] and a bearer of divine wisdom he hadn't shared with his male followers.

Fortunately, fragments of the Gospel of Mary survived and were unearthed in the late 19th century. It's the only early Christian gospel written in the name of a woman. And her words are revolutionary. Mary's gospel insists that we are not full of sin, but inherently good. She reminds us that the kingdom of heaven isn't a distant place to achieve in the afterlife but a reality already within us. 'The kingdom is here,' she says, 'but you do not see it.'

Her most radical teaching, 'What is within you will save you,' tells us that salvation isn't something we need earn or have granted by an external force. The 'ascension' we're all here to undertake isn't a joyride up to heaven but an inward journey. One that leads to our truest self. Therefore, the power we seek is already inside us. All we need to do is wake up – to become more present.[10]

Healing isn't about becoming someone new or proving yourself worthy to someone or something external – it's about returning to who you've always been.

No matter your faith or whether you follow one at all, Mary Magdalene's gospel remains profoundly relevant. It teaches us that we don't need to look outward for rescue, only inward. It calls us to reclaim what patriarchy tried to strip away: our inner sanctuary. Divinity has always been alive within us.

I hypothesize that male-centric religions were created not as a divine truth but as a deflection – an attempt to mask the envy and discomfort that arises from the undeniable power women carry in their bodies. The power to create, to nourish, to sustain life, and perceive imbalance.

And instead of revering that mystery, they tried to control it. They feared it. The early Christian Church, for example, was deeply invested in a strictly patrilineal narrative: Jesus, born of God in heaven, assembled an all-male circle of disciples and, upon his ascension, passed authority to them – period.

They positioned themselves as the origin point of divine order and cast women as the derivative, conveniently ignoring the fact that every human, prophet or not, came first through the body of a woman.

The Sanctuary of Safety

As we near the conclusion of this first part of the journey, one undeniable truth stands clear: Women do not feel safe within patriarchal systems. Not safe to be themselves, to express their truth, to chase success sustainably; not safe to trust their instincts, have their symptoms heard, inhabit their bodies, rest without guilt, or even move freely through the world.

Whether it's dealing with sexual harassment at work, walking home at night with keys clenched between your fingers, facing online abuse or harassment, being denied access to reproductive rights, or navigating life outside the gender binary – the message is clear: *You're not safe here.*

But as you began to see by learning about how your hormones work, the danger doesn't stop at the external forces. The systems we've explored have been internalized. They live in our cells, our breath, our cycles, our emotional responses. They shape how we interpret stress, how our hormones function, and how our nervous system responds to life itself.

At the heart of it all is the most fundamental question your body asks, moment by moment: *Am I safe, or am I unsafe?* This binary, unconscious calculation is the hidden operating system behind so much of what we experience. But just as Mary taught us, no matter how loud the world gets or how much chaos surrounds us, there's a deeper truth we can return to. Safety is something we can restore within.

...

Now that you're beginning to understand how the pressures of patriarchy and chronic stress shape your biology, it's time to shift gears and talk about solutions. In the next chapter, you'll be introduced to my Root Restoration

Framework – a healing model that bridges the external systems we've been talking about with your internal response to them. This is where we move from awareness to action, and begin the process of reclaiming your safety, balance, and power from the inside out.

Chapter 8
INTRODUCING THE ROOT RESTORATION FRAMEWORK

'What is your inside is your outside.'

THE THUNDER, PERFECT MIND 4:30–31

The vital importance of restoring a sense of internal safety didn't occur to me in one singular moment. It was something I had to learn through lived experience, over and over again, as my health unraveled and I looked for answers from two different worlds.

In one world stood my father: a brilliant physician grounded in the evidence-based rigor of Western medicine and publishing in prestigious journals such as *The New England Journal of Medicine* and *The Lancet*. In the other was my mother: a self-described 'rule-breaker' who refused to submit to a lifetime of medication for her autoimmune condition, bringing her body into remission through a fusion of Western medicine, Eastern wisdom, holistic practices, and major lifestyle changes.

When I began falling apart at age 12 – experiencing period pain, migraines, anxiety, eczema, peeling skin, digestive issues, even life-threatening anaphylaxis – my parents did all they could to find solutions. Western doctors analyzed me in pieces: one symptom and prescription at a time. While my mother took me to practitioners who asked: 'What's your body trying to say? What's this pain protecting you from? What are you holding inside?'

I found value in both approaches – Western medicine offered structure and intervention, while holistic traditions spoke to something deeper, more intuitive. But I couldn't yet find a way to bring them together. And despite having access to every resource imaginable, I was still told I'd likely never have children and that I'd be managing chronic symptoms for life.

Reclaiming Our Inner Safety and Power

My health didn't improve in a sustained or meaningful way until my transformative year at Timbertop, which I described in Chapter 3. But when the COVID-19 lockdowns hit, from 2020, I fell apart again, this time more intensely. My hair started thinning dramatically. My face was swollen, my belly constantly bloated, and coarse hairs began growing under my chin. I developed body dysmorphia from the constant changes, digestive distress, and a growing sense that I was a stranger inside my own skin.

On paper, I was doing everything right – eating well, moving my body, getting adequate sleep, and meditating. But the problem didn't lie in what I was *doing* but in how I was *feeling*. It was internal.

That's when I began to understand that no amount of lab tests or supplements can compensate for a life lived out of alignment with who you really are. If your daily choices betray your values, your truth, your cyclical blueprint, or emotional safety, your body will sound the alarm.

I'd become a woman shaped by systems: high achieving, disciplined, and validated through approval, but disconnected from my inner voice. I wore my diagnoses and burnout like badges of honor, hoping someone – some system – would swoop in and save me. I finally learned that healing doesn't come from being rescued. It comes from reclaiming yourself. If I wanted to truly heal, I had to take radical responsibility for both my external and internal worlds.

So, I began to track not just my physical symptoms but also the deeper behavioral and relational patterns (the unconscious dynamics, roles, and responses we repeat in relationships, often shaped by past experiences, trauma, or unmet needs) that had shaped my life. With each step, I identified and then pruned the roots that had kept me stuck and learned to honor my body.

Sixteen years after my first painful period, I'd not only completely reversed my PCOS – even healing the cysts on my ovaries – but also restored my digestion, lost stubborn weight, grown longer, healthier hair, transformed my skin, and reclaimed my mental health.

With my newfound energy and clarity, I also made profound shifts in my relationships and career. I'd finally found a path that aligned with my authentic desires and deepest purpose. This was no longer just healing – it was a complete reclamation of my power.

The Root Restoration Framework and ThetaSomatics

That transformation became the foundation for a healing model that I now call the Root Restoration Framework, which integrates modern science, ancient wisdom, and lived experience. While nutrition, lifestyle, and supplementation played an important role by reducing the amount of 'stress' my body was under, I came to understand that true healing involves more than just reducing the load – it requires restoring the body's ability to *carry* it.

> *Our health, fulfillment, and success are shaped by one thing: our nervous system's capacity – the body's ability to feel safe, both psychologically and physiologically.*

Once this clicked, I immersed myself in the science of the nervous system, trauma, and subconscious reprogramming. What emerged was ThetaSomatics™ – my multidimensional approach to building nervous system resilience, restoring hormonal harmony, and rewiring the subconscious mind by releasing stored stress, processing emotional memory, and replacing limiting beliefs with empowered truths; in Part III, we'll be using ThetaSomatics tools to help ease your symptoms.

Inspired by the African proverb 'When roots are deep, there is no need to fear the wind,' the Root Restoration Framework takes the form of a tree. Because safety isn't static – it's a dynamic state, a living foundation. The framework is about cultivating confidence in your physiological and psychological capacity, so that you can face the blows of life's challenges with resilience. It's also about taking full accountability and responsibility for yourself rather than building walls to shield yourself from every possible threat.

When the optimal conditions for the health of a tree are met, flowers and leaves bloom, fruit emerges, and new life is created. The path to reclaiming your power is no different. You, too, were designed to bloom when the conditions are right.

When farmers experience a failed harvest, they don't blame the plants. They examine the environment and ask: *Was there sufficient rainfall? Did the soil hold enough nutrients? Were external factors interfering with growth?* Then they do their best to adjust the ecosystem to create a different outcome.

But when it comes to our own healing, we haven't been taught to ask questions like *What toxins am I exposed to? Do I feel safe to be myself in this environment? What beliefs have dictated my choices?* Instead, we internalize blame or normalize our pain.

Uncovering the Root Cause of Your Symptoms

Ultimately, the Root Restoration Framework is a way back to yourself, to your inner sanctuary. To your power. The illustration below shows its first stage, identifying the deeper patterns beneath our visible symptoms; we'll be working with the second stage in Part III.

Here's an overview of what the Root Restoration tree represents:

- **The branches** of the tree are our *visible symptoms*: the physical, emotional, behavioral, and relational struggles that tend to catch our attention first. These are what we try to manage, suppress, or fix. But too often, they become the sole focus of our efforts, distracting us from what lies beneath.

- **The roots** of the tree are *the root cause* of our visible symptoms: a lack of safety in the body and mind. Until we address the deeper forces that drive and sustain what we're experiencing, real healing will remain out of reach.

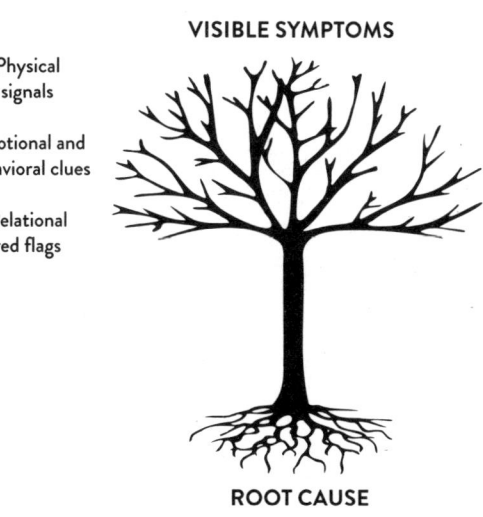

The Root Restoration Framework

Let's now bring the framework to life. The Root Restoration tree shows you how your visible symptoms, the branches, are connected to a deeper root cause: a disruption in your body's sense of safety. The following exercise is a practical tool drawn directly from this model. It's your opportunity to identify the branches that are showing signs of distress or imbalance.

Self-Assessment: How Safe Do You Feel?

This exercise is the first active step in the Root Restoration work you'll continue in Part III, and it's designed to help you start to transform your perception of stress and life's painful experiences into embodied wisdom and strength. You'll reflect not only on your physical symptoms but also on emotional, behavioral, and relational patterns that reveal how safe your mind and body truly feel.

This is the essence of Root Restoration work. When symptoms arise, a powerful woman will ask herself two questions: *What are these symptoms saying about my past and present? What are these symptoms here to teach me for the future?*

Before moving into the self-assessment, I encourage you to take a moment to pause. Notice what you're feeling about your sense of safety. And while you're completing the exercise, if any blame, shame, anger, or guilt surface, know that these emotions hold energy. And that energy can be acknowledged, metabolized, and redirected into aligned action.

Visible Symptoms

Grab a pen or a pencil, settle in, and move through the checklist of symptoms below, ticking off all those that apply to you. Be aware that this isn't about diagnosing yourself – it's about reconnecting with your body's messages and creating space for meaningful change.

Physical Signals

- ☐ Hormonal disruptions (irregular or painful periods, PCOS, PMS, PMDD, or endometriosis symptoms)
- ☐ Adrenal issues (cortisol dysregulation, burnout)
- ☐ Sleep disturbances (insomnia or trouble sleeping)
- ☐ Weight fluctuations (unexplained gain/loss or difficulty losing weight)
- ☐ Digestive issues (bloating, IBS-like symptoms, poor nutrient absorption)
- ☐ Skin flare-ups (acne, eczema, or other inflammatory skin conditions)
- ☐ Chronic tension (jaw clenching, neck and shoulder tension, back or hip pain, migraines, pelvic floor tightness or pain)
- ☐ Emotional and mental distress (anxiety, OCD tendencies, panic episodes, low or depressive moods)
- ☐ Autoimmune-related symptoms (chronic inflammation, joint pain, fatigue, or flare-ups linked with conditions such as Hashimoto's, lupus, or rheumatoid arthritis)

Emotional and Behavioral Clues

- ☐ Persistent low self-worth or feelings of inadequacy
- ☐ Overwhelmingly negative self-talk ('I'm not enough' narratives)
- ☐ Compulsive people-pleasing ('I must make others happy')
- ☐ Perfectionism, overachievement, and hyper-responsibility (believing that worth is tied to productivity)
- ☐ Difficulty expressing or processing anger (repressing self-protective emotions or believing 'I can't control my emotions')
- ☐ Controlling behaviors as a mechanism to create the illusion of safety (includes overplanning and micromanaging to feel secure, although that often fuels anxiety and limits flexibility)

- [ ] Chronic fear of disappointing others or letting them down

Relational Red Flags

- [ ] Patterns of toxic or unbalanced relationships
- [ ] Overextension in caregiving roles; sacrificing personal well-being
- [ ] Difficulty establishing or maintaining healthy boundaries
- [ ] Believing 'I'm responsible for how others feel'

Most of the women who come to see me about period and reproductive issues recognize themselves in most of these symptoms. So, if you've ticked off a lot of the boxes and feel a flicker of concern rising, reframe it as empowerment. These signs are simply your mind and body communicating with you. And now, perhaps for the first time, you're truly listening.

Root Cause: A Lack of Safety

Your visible symptoms – whether physical, emotional, behavioral, or relational – are rooted in deeper patterns that threaten your internal sense of safety. These often include trauma, unprocessed experiences, limiting beliefs, learned behaviors, and environmental stressors.

In Part II, I'll help you to build on the clarity you've just unlocked here by teaching you how to understand your biology, your hormones, your nervous system, and how your body actually works. Because when you can finally name and understand what's happening inside you, you stop outsourcing your power. You stop trying to fix what was never broken and start partnering with the wisdom that's been there all along.

In Part III, we'll focus on the second stage of the framework – Root Restoration – which will help you to trace your symptoms back to what I call the five core roots of safety. However, by completing this self-assessment, you've already begun the process by bringing awareness to the specific ways your body is asking for restoration. This tool is a chance to witness what's been living under the surface and to reconnect with your body's messages.

From Holding It All to Holding Yourself

It's time to reclaim the role of the healer and nurturer of your own life, stepping into the full force of who you've always been. This is no easy task. For years, often decades, we've been taught to look outward for inner stability and safety. We've leaned on partners, careers, mentors, or institutions to hold us steady, filling in the gaps we weren't taught how to hold for ourselves. We've been raised to believe that safety lies in compliance, performance, and being needed.

Recognizing those patterns and preparing to release them – which we'll be doing in Part II – requires faith in your body's signals. Faith in your intuition. Faith in your ability to discern what's right for you and to stand by it, even if others don't understand.

And that's especially difficult when, like the connective tissue that holds the body together, women have long been expected to hold together everything around them – families, workplaces, communities – often at great personal cost.

It's no coincidence that women are disproportionately affected by conditions impacting connective tissue, such as lupus, fibromyalgia, and rheumatoid arthritis.[1] They're a reflection of the weight we carry. A mirror of the societal expectation that we must bind, support, and stretch ourselves endlessly to keep everyone else intact.

This same insight can be extended to reproductive health issues. Conditions such as PCOS, endometriosis, and infertility reveal what happens when the systems designed to sustain and generate life have been overstretched.

Dr. Gabor Maté, a prominent voice in mind–body medicine, has long observed that those suffering from chronic conditions often share a similar profile: difficulty saying no, a compulsion to meet others' needs, and deeply ingrained perfectionism.[2] Likewise, a 2021 study in *Psychological Medicine*[3] found strong links between chronic stress, perfectionistic traits, and immune dysfunction.

When you look closely, you'll see that these traits are the very behaviors society conditions women to perform from childhood. And because they're so often praised and rewarded, we rarely question them. But they're survival strategies. Habits we inherit in order to feel safe, needed, and loved.

Cultivating a sense of inner safety, then, isn't about rejecting your roles or responsibilities. It's about releasing the belief that they *define* you. It's about unhooking from the identity of the 'good girl,' the perfectionist, and the martyr. Meeting yourself without conditions. Learning to support yourself as fiercely as you've supported everyone else.

...

Now you know that the root cause of your symptoms is a lack of safety in mind and body, the next part of the book will take you into the first phase of the solution. Before you can make meaningful change, you need to understand what's actually happening inside your body and why. Part II will help you decode your body's signals, understand the science behind them, and step into your role as the keeper of your own healing wisdom.

We'll explore the science behind your symptoms, because when you understand your biology, you gain the courage, clarity, and consistency required to meet the world differently. Remember, while you'll never have *control* over the circumstances that life throws your way, you'll always have the power to choose how you *respond* to them.

Part II
THE SYSTEM IN YOUR CELLS

This is where everything changes. Because for the patriarchy, women's widespread ignorance of their own biology is bliss. When we don't understand how our mind and body work, it's easier to dismiss their signals. To internalize the beliefs that we're faulty or defective – too emotional, too sensitive, too much.

But that's not your reality anymore.

This is the part of the book where we turn inward.

We'll explore how external patriarchal systems have been absorbed into your biology, and you'll begin to understand that patterns like people-pleasing, perfectionism, emotional reactivity, chronic fatigue, and even autoimmune flares aren't character flaws – they're survival responses; intelligent adaptations wired into your nervous system in response to stress, trauma, and cultural conditioning.

We'll explore how your health is shaped by your environment and how unresolved emotional experiences and inherited beliefs show up as physical symptoms. You'll start to connect the dots between your lived experience and the messages your body has been trying to send.

With the help of scientific insights and more awareness of the root cause of your symptoms, you'll begin to see that your body has never been the problem – it's been the messenger.

And now that you're listening, the real solution begins.

Chapter 9
STRESS IS MORE THAN WHAT WE'VE BEEN TOLD

*'If you listen to your body when it whispers,
you won't have to hear it scream.'*

CHEROKEE PROVERB

Stress is a word that entered my vocabulary long before I truly understood what it meant. I remember being asked at school, 'How are the classes? Are they hard?' And without hesitation, I sighed and replied, 'Oh, I'm so busy. It's so stressful.' I was only 11, and already I'd absorbed the idea that being overwhelmed was proof of working hard, being important, being good.

I'm not sure where I learned this – from the hard-working adults around me, from TV shows where women rushed around, breathlessly balancing a million responsibilities, or perhaps simply from living in a world that equates stress with the standard way of being. Whatever the source, I understood at a young age that busyness meant worth.

By the time I became an adult, stress had become my default, something to aspire to. If I wasn't stressed out, was I even trying hard enough? If I wasn't exhausted, was I doing enough? I piled more and more onto my plate, convinced that if I could just handle it all, I'd finally be 'enough.' Until my body had enough and told me otherwise.

The Real Definition of Stress

Most of us have been taught to view stress as a villain. Something to conquer, to push through, or even shame ourselves for feeling. But that's the masculine perspective. One that views sensitivity as weakness. The feminine truth is that stress isn't just pressure, it's a signal. An ancient alarm system that warns you something is out of alignment – not just in your calendar, but in your life. Or in the way you're responding to it.

At its best, stress sharpens you. It shows up as nervous energy before your first day in a new job; as a spark of anticipation before a first date; as a warning that something isn't right – that your boundaries are being crossed, or you're being treated unfairly.

And at the other end of the spectrum, stress shows up as the electric charge of sexual attraction – a quickened pulse, a flutter of aliveness, and a pull toward possibility. Chemically, stress and excitement are nearly identical. So, it's your interpretation of stress that's turning tension into terror, or conversely, transformation. This is when stress is at its most constructive. When it's here to awaken and protect you.

As we touched on in Chapter 2, women are far more likely than men to receive a vague diagnosis of 'it's just stress,' often without any deeper investigation. This reflects a broader pattern in healthcare – one that tends to minimize or dismiss women's experiences unless they align with a socially accepted, high-stakes narrative. Stress is only taken seriously when it's linked to something dramatic and visible, such as a job loss, divorce, or the death of a loved one. But this definition of damaging stress is woefully incomplete.

Women from all over the world have come to me saying 'I don't feel stressed.' Confused by their symptoms, they scan their lives for obvious triggers and find none. If there's no major upheaval, no immediate crisis, then surely they must be stress-free. However, there's a hidden truth here:

You don't have to feel stressed to be stressed.

We've been taught that stress is something we feel. Something obvious. But in fact, stress is anything that places strain on your body's systems, whether you're aware of it or not. The stress response has even been measured in the body when someone is unconscious under general anesthetic.[1] Let that sink in for a moment. Your body can be experiencing stress without you consciously being aware of it.

Our Allostatic Load (Stress Bucket)

So, stress isn't just about what you think or feel. It's a deeply ingrained, automatic process that often operates on autopilot as your body works tirelessly to maintain balance. And when the weight of that load exceeds your body's ability to recover, symptoms begin to surface.

As Hans Selye, the endocrinologist who pioneered stress research, revealed in the mid-20th century, it's rarely the singular, catastrophic events that push our bodies to breaking point. Instead, it's the relentless accumulation of our unmet needs, unspoken traumas, and inherited burdens[2] – the invisible 'allostatic load' we carry, so deeply embedded in our lives that it often feels normal.

Stress is an umbrella term that includes both short-term pressures and chronic, systemic forces that quietly accumulate, shaping our health and well-being in ways we often fail to notice. While writing this book, I had the opportunity to speak with Dr. Andrew Neville, an adrenal fatigue specialist who's been studying the stress response for 20 years, and he explained the concept of stress in a clear and simple way:

'I think of each of us as having a stress bucket (allostatic load),' he said. 'This includes physical, mental, emotional, and chemical stress, as well as environmental toxins, infections, injuries, surgeries, poor diet, work, family struggles, divorce, and, of course, trauma. One of the key aspects of healing is creating as much room in the stress bucket as possible.'

Types of Stress

To help my clients better understand how different types of stress contribute to the full allostatic load on the body, I categorize stress into three types. While they coexist and interrelate, they each have their own impact:

- **Shock stress:** These are sudden, short-term stressors that activate the body's stress response. Examples would be an argument with your mother, an impending deadline, public speaking, or a loud bang during the night that startles you awake.

- **Slow-burn stress:** These are chronic, low-grade stressors that quietly deplete your body's resources over time. For example, poor sleep, nutrient deficiencies, environmental toxins, overworking, air pollution, loneliness, or a lack of orgasms.

- **Silent stress:** This is the constant, low-level stress or background hum that quietly accumulates over time. For example, the gender pay gap, the mental load of caregiving, cultural biases, and decades' worth of unprocessed emotions still in your system.

In Part III, the second stage of the Root Restoration Framework will guide you in identifying and releasing all three types of stress. But first, we need to grasp just how deeply stress reshapes us by unpacking the mechanisms of the *stress response*. This sets us up to explore how stress interacts with the nervous system, how trauma rewires our internal landscape, and how unprocessed emotions become embedded in the body.

Understanding the Stress Response

While stress evolved as an adaptive, short-term reaction to a threat, we've become so accustomed to living in this heightened state that it no longer feels like a warning. And when we keep layering on stressors such as multitasking, emotional suppression, under-sleeping, overworking, people-pleasing, and worrying about how we're perceived, the signals get louder.

What begins as low-level irritability or fatigue can evolve into anxiety, gut issues, period problems, skin conditions, and chronic pain. To understand why that happens, we need to get to know the stress response for what it really is – a full-body cascade of biological changes designed to keep us alive.

Acute Stress Response (Fight-or-Flight)

Picture this: You're driving a car along a road when suddenly another vehicle veers into your lane, cutting you off. Your foot slams on the brakes, the tires screech, and your chest tightens. Your heart hammers against your ribcage, and your breath quickens into shallow gulps. That jolt, that visceral rush, is your stress response in full force, mobilizing every resource in your body to shield you from the threat.

Here's what's happening behind the scenes: The moment your nervous system detects a perceived threat, it sends an urgent message to your brain to determine whether a stress response is needed. The hypothalamus, deep in the brain, quickly assesses the situation. Crucially, it doesn't just react to the present moment, it also cross-references stored memories, beliefs, and past experiences.

This means your stress response isn't just based on what's happening now, it's influenced by your history and past encounters with similar situations (there's more on this coming up in the next chapter).

If the hypothalamus perceives danger, it activates the sympathetic nervous system (SNS), which signals the adrenal glands to release stress hormones such as adrenaline (epinephrine) and noradrenaline (norepinephrine). Then, if the threat persists, the hypothalamus engages the hypothalamic-pituitary-adrenal (HPA) axis, leading to the release of cortisol and other supportive stress hormones. These flood your body with the message 'survival mode activated.'

This acute stress response is commonly known as fight-or-flight, which is the body's built-in survival mechanism – a rapid-fire reaction that prepares you to either confront a threat (fight), escape it (flight), or, in some cases, freeze or fawn (more on those in Chapter 10).

Every system in your body shifts into protection mode. Heightened alertness, faster breathing, increased heart rate – responses all designed to keep you alive. And in this state, your body reallocates resources, prioritizing what's necessary for immediate survival and sidelining everything else.

Below are some of the ways fight-or-fight plays out in the body:

- **The digestive system** slows down, often resulting in bloating, cramps, or constipation.
- **Reproductive processes** are paused, leading to irregular cycles, reduced fertility, or loss of libido.
- **The immune system** takes a backseat, leaving us more vulnerable to illness.

As Dr. Neville put it: 'The mistake many patients and practitioners make is chasing these secondary conditions as if they're the root cause rather than recognizing them as symptoms of a broken stress-response system. Trying to fix these problems while still stuck in fight-or-flight is like trying to push a car with the parking brake engaged.'

Chronic Stress Response

When stressors accumulate faster than your body can recover, or when you don't have adequate time to rest your nervous system, the stress response stays activated for longer than it should – shifting stress from a protective force to a predatory one. Cortisol continues to circulate as a long-term disruptor, quietly unravelling balance across the body by throwing the hormone hierarchy off-kilter (*see page 47*) and with it, every major function – digestion, immunity, metabolism, reproductive health. Your body, once finely attuned to cycles of activation and rest, is now locked in a loop of anticipation, adapting not to bursts of stress but to stress as its baseline.

At first, your body might produce higher-than-usual cortisol in response to persistent stress, but over time, your adrenal glands can become exhausted from constant overdrive. As a result, cortisol levels can begin to drop, leaving you feeling drained, fatigued, or even depressed. This sustained drop in cortisol (often diagnosed as 'low cortisol') can make it harder for your body to effectively manage stress, pushing you deeper into the cycle of imbalance.

The Body-Wide Effects of Stress

If you've ever lost your appetite after a heartbreak or felt a migraine coming on after a tense exchange, then you've experienced the truth that Western medicine has taken far too long to acknowledge: Your body feels *everything*.

For centuries, the dominant view in Western medicine has been the body is made up of separate, disconnected systems – each studied in isolation as if they weren't in constant conversation. But science is finally catching up with what women have always experienced: Everything is deeply interconnected.

> *What you think, how you feel, and the state of your body are always in dialogue.*

The field of psychoneuroimmunology – how the nervous system, immune system, and emotional world interact – has confirmed that we're not compartmentalized. In fact, our body is made up of one unified, living system, wired together through a network of chemical and neurological pathways that responds moment by moment to the world around us.

Stress isn't just a mental or emotional state – it's a physiological process that can operate beneath your awareness, silently shaping your health. This means that a single thought, a flash of fear, or an unspoken resentment can ripple through your gut, menstrual cycle, immune system, or energy.

Over time, if you remain in a state of chronic stress, those interconnections naturally lead to imbalances across multiple systems. That's why the Root Restoration Framework includes symptoms as diverse as painful periods, jaw clenching, joint pain, and constipation. They may seem unrelated, but they all trace back to one root cause: unresolved stress in a system that feels unsafe.

Completing the 'Stress Response Cycle'

Here's what most of us were never taught: The stress response doesn't end just because the stressful moment is over. To return to a state of balance where healing can take place, we need to show the body that the event or danger has been resolved.

We see this in animals – consider how a dog trembles during a thunderstorm or how a duck shakes off the tension in its wings after an argument with another duck over a piece of bread. Whether during or just after a stressful event, these behaviors are natural ways of releasing the built-up energy from the stress response, signaling to the animals' bodies that it's time to heal and recover. That it's safe to return to calm.

What do humans do? We usually suppress or avoid fully processing these emotions. We put on a smile and go about our day, even if we're still seething or on edge inside. We believe that once an event is over, we've 'dealt with it.' But stress doesn't just disappear.

If we don't move the emotional charge through our bodies, it lingers. And when these strong emotions aren't processed, they continue to run in the background – like an engine revving long after the race has finished. Completing the stress response cycle through physical or emotional release is essential to restore safety.

To truly break free from chronic stress and reactivity we need to complete the stress response physically by speaking the languages of the body: movement, breath, and sensation. You'll be guided through exercises to do this in Chapter 20.

Whether it's crying, dancing, laughing, hugging a pet, breathing deeply, jumping up and down, exercising, screaming into a pillow, or moving your body in any way that feels good – these actions help signal to your nervous system that the threat is over and it's safe to deactivate the stress response. This is how we begin working with the nervous system to restore safety and release the lingering tension that stress leaves behind.

* * *

While stress is the language your body uses to signal danger, it's your nervous system that decides what's safe, what's threatening, and when to fight, flee, or freeze. In the next chapter, we'll explore the female nervous system and why in the modern world it's especially vulnerable to chronic imbalance.

Chapter 10
UNLOCKING THE SECRETS OF THE FEMALE NERVOUS SYSTEM

'We look for the Secret... and all the time it is carrying us about... It is the human nervous system itself.
ROBERT ANTON WILSON

Before you open your eyes in the morning, before you decide what to wear or check your phone, a part of you has already started navigating the day. It's not your conscious mind. It's something deeper. Something older. This is your body's command center – the nervous system. A vast electrical network that connects every organ, every muscle, every cell, it's always scanning your external and internal environments to ask: *Am I safe, or unsafe?*

It's the nervous system that initiates your stress response and keeps you alive, regulating your breath without you noticing it. It sets the pace of your heart, filters what you perceive as a threat, and determines whether you feel grounded or restless, present or on edge.

The nervous system governs every aspect of your experience – from your digestion to your sleep, from your choice in romantic partner to the way you respond in a difficult conversation. It's not just another system inside of you – it *is* you.

However, the human nervous system evolved in the Stone Age world, where survival depended on split-second decisions, threats were rare but immediate, and people ran from danger and then rested, allowing the body to return to balance. It wasn't designed for our world, where there's constant pressure to do more, be more, produce more.

And although we've developed advanced cognitive abilities since our nervous system was established, such as abstract thought, problem-solving, and self-awareness, the system is still running on ancient and binary programming language. Deep within us, primal neural circuits remain hardwired, governing the foundational survival responses we share with other mammals: fight-or-flight and freeze.

The Nervous System 101

The American architect and designer Richard Saul Wurman claimed that a single edition of *The New York Times* contains more information than Shakespeare would have encountered in his entire lifetime.[1] Whether or not that's hyperbole, it cuts to a deeper truth: We're overwhelmed by input.

Every moment, your nervous system is filtering an avalanche of stimuli – texts, headlines, notifications, emotional undercurrents, unspoken expectations. It doesn't pause to evaluate what's essential and what's just noise.

When I finally understood how critical it was to work on my nervous system and take control of my stress response, I followed all the traditional advice – during lockdown, I set firmer boundaries with my housemates, committed to meditation, stacked my morning routine, and practiced breathwork and daily journaling – and I tried all the nervous system regulation tools that promised balance and ease.

For a while, it seemed to work. But eventually, the cracks began to show. I'd feel calm and open in the morning but completely overwhelmed and contracted by lunchtime. I was doing everything 'right,' yet I was still stuck in the same self-soothing behavioral loops such as binge eating. Why? Well firstly, I was using a nervous system approach designed for men.

How the Nervous System Works

Before we dive into the differences between the nervous system in males and females, let's first clarify how it functions. Your nervous system is a vast communication network made up of different branches. One of these is the autonomic nervous system (ANS), which runs automatically in the background, regulating your stress responses, energy, and internal balance. It has two main parts: the sympathetic nervous system (SNS) and the parasympathetic nervous system (PNS). Another important branch is the enteric nervous system (ENS), which lives in the gut and plays a key role in how we process emotion and stress. We'll explore that in more depth shortly.

Now imagine that your nervous system is a car with an automatic gearbox, shifting gears without you consciously controlling it. It adjusts in real time, responding to stressors, regulating your energy, and keeping you alive.

Autonomic Nervous System (ANS) – Gearbox

The autonomic nervous system shifts you between fight-or-flight (sympathetic nervous system, SNS) or rest-and-digest (parasympathetic nervous system, PNS) responses as needed, just like the car automatically adjusting gears to handle speed and braking.

Sympathetic Nervous System (SNS) – Accelerator

Press the accelerator, and the car surges forward. That's your SNS in action, activating the stress response to keep you alert, ready, and reactive. Your body reallocates resources to prioritize what's immediately necessary for survival.

Parasympathetic Nervous System (PNS) – Brake

Tap the brakes, and the car slows down. This is your rest, digest, and recovery mode, the state where healing and self-repair happens. The PNS lowers your heart rate, restores digestion, regulates your hormone levels, and brings you back to balance after stress so you can focus on repairing any damage.

Enteric Nervous System (ENS) – Second Brain

The ENS is a vast network of more than 100 million neurons embedded in the walls of our gastrointestinal tract, stretching from the esophagus to the rectum – which is why our gut is often called the 'second brain.' While the ENS can function independently, it's in constant communication with the ANS through the vagus nerve, which extends from our gut, through our heart and lungs, all the way up to our face and ear canal into our brain.

The Gut–Brain Connection

This is why stress hits the gut so hard – when the SNS is in overdrive, digestion slows, leading to bloating, constipation, or nausea. On the flip side, when you're relaxed (in the PNS), digestion flows effortlessly.

One of my clients, who's in her fifties, spent more than a decade struggling with severe constipation every time she stayed with her in-laws over the holiday season. Her gut wasn't malfunctioning – her body simply didn't feel safe enough in that environment to let go. The lesson here is that your gut isn't just reacting to what's on your plate – it's reacting to *your life*.

This gut–brain connection was obvious to us long before modern science confirmed it. Think about how we describe emotions in everyday language: *I have a gut feeling about this.* (Your intuition lives in your gut.) *I'm so nervous,*

I could pee my pants. (Stress alters digestion and elimination.) *I'm sh*tting myself.* (Fear makes your bowels move faster.)

What we casually call a 'gut feeling' is now recognized in neuroscience as a form of neuroception: the body's subconscious ability to detect safety or threat through internal signals before the brain consciously registers them.[2] These signals travel through the gut–brain axis – especially the enteric nervous system and vagus nerve[3] – integrating emotional memory, sensory data, and past experiences into a felt sense of knowing.

The Sneaky Role of Slow-Burn Stressors

Remember in the last chapter when we looked at the stressors that don't necessarily send your body into fight-or-flight but still chip away at your resilience over time? One of the ways they do this is by disrupting your gut health and weakening your ENS.

Unlike an argument, stressors such as ultra-processed foods, chronic sleep deprivation, environmental toxins, recreational drugs, and certain medications don't always cause a dramatic spike in cortisol. Instead, they create a slow, insidious form of stress – chronic inflammation and an imbalance in gut bacteria that disrupts the way the ENS communicates with the brain, reducing the body's ability to shift out of a stress response (SNS) and into a state of recovery (PNS) and weakening our ability to trust our gut instinct.[4]

And here's where it becomes a vicious cycle: The stress response itself also alters your gut bacteria, which in turn weakens the body's ability to handle future stress.[5] This bidirectional relationship means that in order to cultivate internal safety, you need a holistic approach that handles all types of stressors, restoring balance from the inside out (like the one you'll start using in Part III). Remember, stress isn't just about what happens *to you*; it's about what your body can handle.

Nervous System Regulation

A healthy nervous system naturally moves fluidly between activation (fight-or-flight) and recovery (rest and digest) as needed. That's what we call nervous system regulation – the ability to move fluidly between activation and recovery. To meet the moment and then return to safety.

In this state, your body is adaptable, resilient, and capable of healing. You think clearly, rest deeply, and respond to life with intention. But when your system becomes overwhelmed by chronic stress, trauma, inflammation, or unprocessed emotion this balance breaks down. And that's called dysregulation: when your nervous system gets stuck in a chronic state of activation even when the immediate threat has passed.

Dysregulation can look like anxious agitation, burnout, hypervigilance, exhaustion, brain fog, numbness, emotional reactivity, or the emergence of physical symptoms. The good news is that nervous system regulation is a skill anyone can learn. And the more you understand the mechanisms behind it (the physiology of safety and survival), the more power you have to influence your state.

The practices you'll meet in Part III are designed to restore nervous system regulation by working with your body in the languages it understands. And once you know how to return to internal safety, everything changes: your resilience and confidence, your hormones, your cycles, your immune system, your relationships and sense of self.

The Role of the Brain

Now, you might be thinking, *I thought the brain was the body's command center.* Well – plot twist – the latest science suggests the brain isn't the all-powerful CEO we once thought. It's more like a logistics warehouse. In fact, only 20 percent of your body's signals travel from the brain down to the body, but 80 percent travel from the body up to the brain.[6]

In other words, your body is speaking to your brain far more than your brain is speaking to your body. The signals move up and down the vagus nerve, which is constantly sending updates between your body and brain. It's not a top-down hierarchy where your brain is barking orders at your body. Instead, brain and body are deeply intertwined, woven together by the nervous system like an intricate feedback loop.

*Your mind lives in your body,
and your body shapes your mind.*

Now you can understand why telling yourself to 'just relax' or 'stop overreacting' doesn't work. You can't outthink a system that's hardwired to feel first and think later. To truly shift out of stress and downregulate from the SNS to the PNS, you need to speak your body's language. That's where the real magic happens, and we'll continue diving deeper into that in the coming chapters.

But let's return to the key role your brain *does* play: helping your nervous system to react quickly to danger by pulling from past experiences, traumas, and subconscious beliefs in your limbic system. The oldest and most instinctual part of your brain, the limbic system, doesn't analyze; it simply reacts. Bypassing your newer, more evolved and logical brain (the prefrontal cortex) to send the message that it's time to flood your system with stress hormones.

Because this system evolved long before your rational brain did, it cannot distinguish real danger from perceived danger. Your body just can't tell the difference between a physical threat (like being chased by a bear) and an emotional one (such as feeling embarrassed during a meeting). It doesn't pause to analyze whether the danger is real, imagined, immediate, or minor. It just hits the panic button.

How the Nervous System Learns

The nervous system is so foundational to our survival that it begins developing in the womb before our heart starts beating, setting the tone for how we'll navigate the world. But here's the fascinating part: It doesn't just develop, it listens. Becoming fluent in a language far more ancient than words: the language of safety.

In the womb, our nervous system is absorbing cues about safety, stress, and nourishment through our mother's body: her hormonal state, her stress levels, the rhythm of her heartbeat. These are the first messages our nervous system receives about the environment we're about to enter.

It decides, at the most primal level, whether we're being born into a world where it's safe to relax and grow or whether we need to brace for survival. For some, this means being wired for calm and connection. For others, it means being primed for hypervigilance in a world that feels uncertain, unpredictable, or unsafe.

The moment we leave the womb, light, sound, temperature shifts, and separation from our mother introduce entirely new sensations, and our nervous system scrambles to make sense of them. Unlike in the womb, where nourishment and warmth were automatic, survival now depends on external cues – on whether a caregiver picks us up when we cry, on whether comfort comes reliably or unpredictably.

If our early environment is stable – if we're soothed, held, and met with warmth – our nervous system wires for safety. It learns that stress is temporary, and that discomfort is followed by relief. But if care is inconsistent, if stress is prolonged or unresolved, our nervous system adjusts to this unpredictability, bracing for survival rather than settling into ease.

This process isn't unique to any one person: It's part of being human. But for women, the stakes are different. Over the next two chapters we'll explore how trauma disrupts this process, rewiring our bodies for survival in ways that are often invisible but deeply felt. But now that we've got the basics of the nervous system down, let's explore the secrets of the female nervous system.

Female vs. Male Nervous System

Unsurprisingly, the science of the nervous system has been studied largely through a male lens. However, emerging research is starting to show that there are significant differences in the ways that women need to cultivate inner safety and nervous system regulation.

The female nervous system is biologically attuned to connection, shaped by cyclical hormonal fluctuations and influenced by a complex interplay of neurochemicals. In contrast to the stress-and-reward cycles observed in men, its more relationally responsive, with oxytocin – the hormone linked to love, connection, bonding, safety, and restoration – acting as a powerful buffer against stress and a key modulator of nervous system regulation.

This is why the dominant tools and practices for nervous system regulation – designed around male physiology – often fall short for women. They're linear, performance-based, dopamine-driven: Set and achieve clear goals, build rigid routines, push through discomfort, achieve through repetition, and cultivate resilience through endurance.

> *Women aren't designed to grind in a straight line toward success, endlessly producing, performing, and competing. We're designed to ebb and flow. To adapt, receive, reflect.*

When women regulate through dopamine alone, they experience high highs and low lows (exhaustion disguised as productivity); over-reliance on external validation (seeking proof of worth through work); and chronic shame and self-criticism (feeling they're 'too much' or 'not enough').

The Functional Freeze Response

Women are conditioned to believe that the acts that restore us – pausing, receiving, and softening – are indulgent, lazy, or even shameful. But they're none of these things – they are biological imperatives. When we're denied these essential rhythms, when oxytocin is chronically depleted, we don't just get tired, we slip into functional freeze, the most insidious of the nervous system's survival strategies.

Functional freeze isn't the visible panic of fight-or-flight, the rush of adrenaline, or the edge of hypervigilance. It's the slow, silent shutdown of a woman who's become disconnected from herself. She keeps moving, keeps producing, keeps achieving, but inside, there's a numbness, a sense of estrangement from her own body and desires.

Functional freeze often shows up as chronic fatigue, emotional numbness, overworking to avoid feelings, and perfectionism to maintain control. This is why we're witnessing the end of the 'boss babe' era and the ushering-in of the 'soft girl' age – a cultural reckoning where women are realizing that slowing down is what will actually allow them to speed up.

The Fawn Response

But what happens when women turn outward in search of safety? This points to another evolutionary adaptation in the female nervous system: the 'tend-and-befriend' response. Deeply influenced by oxytocin, this ensured the survival of not just the individual but the entire group.

But when true, nourishing connection isn't available, this drive can morph into something more precarious – the fawn response. Instead of forming authentic bonds, women may begin to over-accommodate, people-please, or sacrifice their own needs to maintain a sense of safety. What begins as a natural, life-affirming impulse toward community becomes a survival mechanism rooted in appeasement and self-abandonment.

In this state, women may look connected, but inwardly, they're trapped in a cycle of *performing* safety rather than truly *feeling* it. And while this may initially stave off discomfort, over time it leads to the same disconnection we see in functional freeze: a life lived on the surface, disconnected from the deeper pulse of our own authentic wants, needs, and desires.

Oxytocin: Sustainer of Life

The hormone oxytocin has been shaping us for more than 200 million years – when mammals first emerged, it became the biochemical foundation of bonding, communication, and survival. The ability to feel closeness, trust, and love is deeply biological and hundreds of studies now confirm that oxytocin plays a major role in managing stress and regulating pain. Ancient cultures knew this intuitively and prioritized female nervous system regulation practices such as women's circles and fertility rituals that kept women grounded.

Your relationships are one of the most powerful of the forces that shape the state of your nervous system, which is why it's important to choose them wisely. Our nervous system was not designed to function in isolation but to thrive in safe, supportive connections where love and care could shift our internal filters, constantly reminding us that we're safe. Without adequate oxytocin, our life force energy and nervous system capacity slowly wither away.

> *Oxytocin is the body's way of communicating to each woman:*
> *'You're safe. You belong. You're needed. You're held.'*

This is why we crave synchronized group activities like Pilates, yoga, and dance classes; why we join book clubs and eagerly anticipate long brunches with friends; why talking to a best friend can instantly shift your mood; and why a long, heartfelt hug is often the best remedy after a hard day at work. All these things recreate the nervous system regulation we once found in communal movement and ritual. Our bodies are trying to tell us that healing happens in togetherness.

The resurgence of 'girlhood' culture – Taylor Swift concerts, the *Barbie* and *Wicked* movies, the rise of 'hot girl walks,' self-care rituals, BookTok and book clubs – reflects women's universal, instinctual need for community and the healing power of oxytocin.

How to Boost Your Oxytocin Levels

Here are some more ways to consciously increase your ability to make and use oxytocin. How many of these behaviors and activities are already a regular part of your life? Are you lacking some of them? Do you find yourself finding ways to resist or put off the urge to do things like this? How can you welcome more oxytocin into your life?

- **Touch and physical connection** (hugs, intimacy, affectionate gestures)
- **For mothers: breastfeeding and nurturing bonds** (deep connection, nourishment, attunement)
- **Orgasm and somatic release** (letting go, relaxation, nervous system reset)
- **Relational safety and co-regulation** (being seen and heard in our authenticity)
- **True sisterhood and support** (women's circles, collaboration over competition)
- **Receiving and allowing** (letting in love, help, and abundance without guilt)
- **Sacred rituals and celebration** (honoring life phases, menstrual cycles, transitions)

- **Nature and embodiment** (connecting with the Earth and coming back into your body through sunlight, gentle movement, breath, grounding, and sensory presence – fully inhabiting the here and now)
- **Laughter, play, and joy** (expression, spontaneity, and ease without shame)
- **Storytelling and creative expression** (dancing, singing, and speaking our truth)

We're being called to let go of guilt and embrace what nourishes us, unlocking our body's capacity to heal and expanding our nervous system's capacity.

The Impact of the Menstrual Cycle

Another key feature of the female nervous system is its dynamic relationship with the menstrual cycle. As every woman experiences, different phases of the cycle don't just affect our hormones, they influence how we feel, think, respond, and recover.

You might notice you're more outgoing and energized one week, and more sensitive or withdrawn the next. One moment you're breezing through life, the next you're crying over a text or feeling inexplicably overwhelmed by the simplest tasks.

This isn't in your head. It's in your hormones. Shifts in estrogen, progesterone, and cortisol levels directly impact your nervous system's resilience. At certain points in your cycle, you can handle more. At others, your body's asking you to slow down and receive more support.

What shifts throughout the month is your baseline capacity. In ovulation, your nervous system is more naturally regulated and resilient – meaning you may feel more grounded, energized, or open. But even then, life, relationships, or unresolved trauma can still trigger dysregulation.

Align Your Cycle and Your Nervous System

Learning to work with your cycle and your nervous system together is so powerful: It gives you the capacity to meet each phase with awareness. This is how you become the woman who knows how to manage her energy, emotions, and needs in any season. Let's break this down.

Ovulation/Summer

Your nervous system leans into parasympathetic activation (rest and digest) when you're at peak fertility, which allows you to handle more stress and intensity with ease[7] – for example, going on dates, networking, socializing, pitching at work, running big meetings, and tackling the tasks you've been avoiding.

But there's more to this state than just performance. Relaxation is a prerequisite for libido, and libido is a pathway to orgasm (and oxytocin!). When your body feels safe, your desire can rise. Your tissues soften. Your sensitivity increases. You become more available to pleasure and connection, both with yourself and with others.

Luteal (Premenstrual)/Autumn

The luteal phase is where many women begin to unravel. The nervous system leans toward sympathetic activation (fight-or-flight)[8, 9] so our sensitivity to stress increases, meaning our nervous system needs more resources to stay regulated – more alone time, more nourishment, less external stimulation.

Essentially, the body reacts more strongly to stress during this phase. For neurodivergent women and those with sensory sensitivities, these shifts may be even more pronounced, which makes nervous system support all the more essential.

Your tolerance for BS also drops, which can feel like radical clarity or complete chaos – you either see what's not working in your life or you feel completely overwhelmed by it. Suddenly, your body may feel foreign, your friendships draining, your career a trap. The things you could tolerate last week? Unbearable. The patterns you ignored? Blindingly obvious.

If your nervous system is already taxed, this is the phase where rage, exhaustion, and dysregulation surface as severe PMS, Premenstrual Dysphoric Disorder (PMDD), or even full freeze/shutdown.

Learning to Love Your Cycle

But it doesn't have to be that way. When you start working with your nervous system through the practices I share in Part III, you will build the capacity to hold this intensity with more grace and resilience. And the luteal (premenstrual) phase becomes a time of discernment, boundary-setting, and fierce clarity.

Appreciating these shifts is crucial because how we perceive and emotionally respond to our menstrual cycle can either ease or heighten the stress we experience.[10] Research shows that viewing our periods as a burden or a weakness exacerbates stress responses during the luteal phase, making it harder for the body to recover effectively.

On the other hand, seeing our cycle as a natural, empowering part of life, with natural energy fluctuations, helps reduce stress and supports the nervous system's resilience.[11] Essentially, if you love your cycle, it will love you right back.

⋯

Once I finally stopped trying to out-discipline my dysregulated nervous system and started listening to what it actually needed, my baseline capacity steadied and I was so much calmer. However, I was still easily derailed. What I hadn't yet addressed were the invisible operating instructions my nervous system was still running on: the memories, beliefs, and survival strategies it had learned long ago.

This is the missing piece for so many women. You can calm your nervous system, work with the fluctuations of your menstrual cycle, and build capacity, but if trauma is still defining what your body perceives as 'safe' or 'unsafe,' you'll keep recreating the same patterns no matter how much work you've done.

The good news is that you have the power to change that. You can teach your body a new definition of safety by changing the instructions it's running on. Instructions rooted in who you are *now*, not what you had to do to survive.

In the next chapter, we'll explore how trauma disrupts our two core biological needs – attachment and authenticity – and why so many of the behavioral and relational patterns we struggle with today began as strategies to survive disconnection.

Chapter 11
THE TRAUMA WE DON'T SEE

'Trauma is a fact of life. It does not,
however, have to be a life sentence.'

PETER LEVINE SOCRATES

For many years, I didn't question the story I'd been told about trauma – that the term should be reserved for the catastrophic, the extreme, the headline-worthy. My paternal grandmother's history was the benchmark: surviving World War II concentration camps, immigrating to Australia from Hungary at just 15, overcoming language barriers and prejudice to build a life for her family.

In comparison, my life was comfortable. I had a loving family, a stable childhood. Suggesting that I might carry wounds of my own felt like an insult to my grandmother's sacrifices, a dismissal of her suffering. Even my parents bristled when I began to explore the idea. How could I claim trauma when I'd been given so much?

But trauma isn't just the story of what happened *to* us – it's the story of what happened *inside* us when we didn't feel safe (physically, psychologically, or emotionally). And when I finally allowed myself to widen the lens, to see trauma not as the exception but as the rule, I realized how deeply it's woven into the fabric of all our lives.

For women, trauma isn't just personal: it's systemic, ancestral. It's in the ways we've been conditioned to shrink, play nice, and self-silence. It's in our DNA, passed down through maternal inheritance and etched into our bodies like invisible scars. Our bodies are a record of what's been endured, of pain dismissed as hysteria, of symptoms ignored. The stories of our grandmothers, our mothers, and ourselves are interwoven, each generation carrying the imprint of the last.

The Silent Scripts We Live By

In November 2024, fresh from the rapid completion of my first book and about to begin this one, I was craving something more than just rest – I needed renewal. I was seeking sisterhood, nature, oxytocin, and a reset for my nervous system.

A friend recommended a retreat in the mountains north of Barcelona, Spain, and in my depleted state, I signed up immediately. I didn't read the fine print. I didn't even care about the itinerary. All I needed was a remote setting, nourishing food, and a chance to exhale. This seemed to tick all the boxes.

The first few days were heavenly and unfolded gently: slow mornings with yoga, herbal tea, and smoothie bowls; deep conversations with women I felt like I'd known forever. I could feel the tension in my body begin to melt, the constant hum of stress quieting for the first time in months. But beneath the surface, there was a quiet charge. We were building up to something; I just didn't know what. And then, on our penultimate night, under the glow of a full moon, a group of us crawled into a *temazcal* – a low, dome-shaped hut wrapped in thick blankets.

The word *temazcal* derives from a word in the Native American language, *Nahuatl*, meaning 'house of heat,' but that barely captures the intensity of the experience. Packed tightly together, our bodies slick with sweat, the air thick with steam and the scent of herbs hanging from the ceiling, we sat in the dark. Naked. Vulnerable. Raw.

Our guide, a woman in her sixties with an effortless authority, spoke with a resonance that bypassed the mind and landed directly in the body. She explained that the ceremony would unfold in four stages, each representing an element and a phase of life. When the door to the hut opened after each stage to let in some cool air, it signified the release of what no longer served us from that phase of our life – the fears, trauma, stories, conditioning, and wounds.

The *temazcal*, I learned, is a rite of passage, a spiritual rebirth. 'The first 25 years of life are spent in absorption,' our guide told us. 'You're shaped by your environment – your family, your culture, society's expectations. But at 26, something shifts. You're no longer just a product of what happened to you. You begin to make choices. Not out of survival, not out of programming, but from a place of sovereignty. You own your story.'

Our Identity Is Formed Before We Choose It

Our guide's words echoed what science now confirms about how our brain develops. For the first 25 years of life, the prefrontal cortex – the part responsible for rational thought, discernment, and conscious choice – is still developing. During this time, we aren't shaping our identity as much as absorbing it.

We take in the world around us like a sponge: *Don't touch the hot stove. Look both ways before crossing the road.* Eventually, the messages become more covert: *I have to be perfect to be loved* or *If I express my needs, I'll get in trouble.*

This is especially true in the earliest years of our life. From birth to around the age of seven, we operate primarily in the theta brainwave state – a slow, dreamy frequency that's highly receptive and imaginative. While theta is associated with deep relaxation in adults (commonly accessed during meditation, rhythmic dance, trance, light sleep, or hypnosis), in children it's a natural and dominant state of consciousness.

Theta allows children to absorb information rapidly and intuitively, such as language, emotional patterns, beliefs, and social norms. In theta, we're deeply impressionable. And it's this openness that makes early childhood such a formative time; the subconscious is wide open.

The trade-off, however, is that the subconscious mind absorbs without filtering, recording everything – including cultural bias and emotional absence – as truth. We're not yet choosing who we are. We're being programmed by our caregivers, our communities, and the unspoken rules of our culture.

And so, the foundations of our identity are formed not through conscious choice but through subconscious absorption – through what we repeatedly see, feel, and experience in our environment. These early imprints become the silent scripts we live by until we learn how to meet them with *awareness* – and as we'll explore later in the book, *rewrite* them.

As I sat there in the steaming hut, surrounded by women of all ages from different walks of life, I realized that for all the years I'd spent searching for answers, healing had never been a mystery. It's been with us all along, woven into the rituals, the stories, and wisdom of the women who came before us.

Attachment and Authenticity

Humans are shaped by two core needs: attachment (the need for connection) and authenticity (the need to be who we are). Babies are born profoundly dependent on others. Our motor skills and cognitive abilities are still developing, requiring years of care before we reach even basic self-sufficiency. We're wired for attachment, for connection, from the start, which means that a newborn is biologically dependent on it. From the moment we enter the world, our nervous system attunes to those around us, shaping itself to secure love, approval, and care so that we're fed, kept warm, held, soothed.

Authenticity, meanwhile, is our deep, innate drive to be who we truly are. To express our emotions, needs, and desires without suppression.

For all the ways that trauma is individual, there's one thing that unites nearly all women. Across generations, we've been targeted by a patriarchal culture that, explicitly and implicitly, demeans, distorts, and even impels us to suppress who we are. For most of us, this is the first and deepest wound we experience – the moment our nervous system learns that being fully ourselves isn't always safe.

It starts early. A child senses that her full range of emotions – her anger, sadness, excitement, curiosity – might disrupt the bond with her caregivers, peers, or community, so she does what every nervous system is wired to do: She prioritizes attachment over authenticity. She dims her enthusiasm to avoid being called 'too much.' She holds back her tears so she's not 'too sensitive.' She swallows her anger because 'good girls don't talk back.'

In his book *The Myth of Normal*, Dr. Gabor Maté describes this as 'ground zero for the most widespread trauma in our society.' A trauma so normalized, so woven into the fabric of how we raise girls, that we mistake it for personality rather than adaptation.

The child learns that to belong, certain parts of her must be suppressed. And so, she adapts. She becomes agreeable. And over time, these adaptations solidify into her identity. What started out as survival strategies become the way she moves through the world. She mistakes her programming for personality. And she believes that who she *had* to be to survive, is who she *is*.

The Biology of Loss

Trauma's impact isn't limited to what *did* happen; it also affects what *didn't*. The experiences we *should* have had yet never did. The love that wasn't given, the safety that was missing, the validation for our unique self-expression that never came. This is the concept of the biology of loss – the absence of care, connection, and recognition that can be just as damaging to our mind and body.

> **Pause for Self-Reflection**
>
> Take a moment to think about or journal on the following questions:
>
> - Did you feel truly seen and understood as a child?
> - Were your emotions welcomed, or were you taught to suppress them?
> - Did you feel safe to express yourself authentically, or did you learn that love had conditions?

This kind of loss doesn't feel or look like trauma in the traditional sense. There's no defining moment, no clear wound to point to. Just a lingering belief that something's missing. Or worse, that there's something wrong with you. Healing, then, requires filling in the spaces where you were never fully held, seen, and loved for who you are: completely unique and irreplicable.

The Trauma Spectrum

Every experience in life has the power to shape how you perceive safety, trust, connection, and self-expression. A devastating betrayal? Yes, that leaves a mark. But so does the slow, quiet erosion of self-worth when you're repeatedly overlooked, ignored, or belittled.

Every experience that shapes your sense of safety, identity, and self-worth falls somewhere on the trauma spectrum. Below is a checklist of experiences on this spectrum, grouped into 'Big T' and 'little t' traumas. All of them matter and all of them count.

Read through the list, and tick off the boxes that resonate with your lived experience. I invite you to go slowly. Before you begin, take a few deep, intentional breaths. Place a hand on your heart or belly. Let your body know: *We're safe to look at this now.*

This is about noticing the moments your system adapted, the places your power got paused, and the roots of the patterns you're ready to rewrite. It's a practice of honoring the brilliance and intelligence of your survival. If you feel the urge to minimize, dismiss, or brush something off as 'not that bad,' pause. That's often where the truth lives. Your nervous system doesn't care how you feel about it now – it cares how you felt about it at the time.

And if emotion rises, let it. You're not regressing by releasing emotions, you're remembering. This is how you begin to take back your power: one truth, one breath, and one brave moment of recognition at a time.

Big T Trauma

- ☐ Severe car accident, natural disaster, or house fire
- ☐ Domestic violence or an abusive relationship
- ☐ Physical assault
- ☐ Witnessing or experiencing a violent crime
- ☐ Near-death experience or severe illness
- ☐ Childbirth trauma (e.g. emergency C-section, medical mistreatment, neonatal intensive-care unit experiences)
- ☐ Racism, sexism, gender discrimination
- ☐ Life-threatening medical diagnosis
- ☐ Childhood neglect or extreme emotional deprivation
- ☐ Experiencing war, political violence, or forced migration
- ☐ Loss of a parent or primary caregiver during childhood
- ☐ Sexual assault, abuse, or rape
- ☐ Growing up in extreme poverty, experiencing food insecurity or homelessness
- ☐ Being trapped in an unsafe environment with no escape (e.g. religious or cult abuse)

Little t Trauma

Emotional and Psychological

- ☐ Growing up in a home where emotions were dismissed or shamed
- ☐ Being told that you're 'too sensitive' or 'too much'
- ☐ Chronic people-pleasing and fear of disappointing others
- ☐ Feeling responsible for a parent's emotions
- ☐ Gaslighting in relationships or in the workplace
- ☐ Bullying at school or at home
- ☐ The death of a pet
- ☐ Having your intuition repeatedly ignored or mocked

Cultural and Gender-Based

- ☐ Being conditioned to put others first and shrink your needs
- ☐ Religious purity culture, body shame, or sex negativity
- ☐ Workplace discrimination, sexual harassment, or being overlooked
- ☐ Being ridiculed for ambition, assertiveness, or setting boundaries
- ☐ Feeling unsafe in public spaces or hyperaware of male dominance

Body

- ☐ Chronic dieting, body shame, or disordered eating patterns
- ☐ Medical gaslighting around period pain, PCOS, endometriosis, or other symptoms
- ☐ Birth-control trauma – dismissal, side effects, or overprescription
- ☐ Fertility struggles, miscarriage, or birth trauma
- ☐ Feeling disconnected from or at war with your body

Relational

☐ Being raised by emotionally unavailable caregivers

☐ Betrayal, infidelity, or emotional abandonment in relationships

☐ Fear of rejection or feeling unworthy of love

☐ Repeated toxic friendships that leave you feeling drained or manipulated

☐ Chronic loneliness or feeling like you never fully belong

Work and Financial

☐ Growing up with financial instability or scarcity

☐ Being underpaid or undervalued, or working in a toxic environment

☐ Burnout from hustle culture or high-pressure careers

☐ Feeling guilt around earning, spending, or taking up space professionally

Notice what resonates, and most importantly, don't gaslight yourself into believing you don't have trauma simply because your experiences don't fit an outdated definition. And if you don't have many memories of your childhood, that's okay too. You don't need to recall the exact memory to begin healing it. If you identified with the relational or behavioral patterns in the self-assessment (*see pages 76–78*), your nervous system is already pointing you toward the truth.

The Nuances of Female Trauma

While trauma may be universal, the way it imprints on the body and mind is deeply shaped by gender. Female trauma has a distinct texture, woven from a complex interplay of biology, social conditioning, and the specific types of harm women are more likely to endure.

Women are twice as likely as men to develop post-traumatic stress disorder (PTSD) – 10 to 12 percent of women versus 4 to 6 percent of men[1] – because the nature of the trauma they endure is different, and because they often experience it at more vulnerable times in their lives.

Men's trauma tends to be external: combat, physical assaults, accidents – events that are often isolated and occur later in life. In contrast, women's trauma is more likely to occur within the context of relationships: intimate partner violence, childhood sexual abuse, coercion, and stalking. These experiences often happen at a younger age, during critical periods of development, which amplifies their psychological and physiological impact.[2]

Sexual assault, in particular, carries one of the highest risks for PTSD, with a lifetime prevalence of 50 percent among women who have experienced it.[3] Unlike other forms of trauma, sexual violence deeply violates a person's sense of safety and trust; often it's committed by someone known to the victim, which compounds the emotional and relational aftermath.

But the impact of trauma doesn't end with what happens to us – it continues in how we carry it. Men are more likely to externalize their pain through aggression, recklessness, or substance abuse. Their trauma seeks release through action, even if it's destructive.[4]

Women tend to turn inward. Their trauma folds in on itself in a way that's quieter but no less damaging. They ruminate, replaying painful memories on a loop. They pull back from the world to avoid further harm. They internalize the belief that their suffering is somehow their fault.[5]

The physiological systems designed to help women connect, regulate, and recover – driven by oxytocin – become disrupted. Instead of finding safety in connection, trauma teaches women that isolation is safer, trapping them in cycles of anxiety, depression, shame, and insomnia.

Your Body Is an Archive

Trauma isn't just emotional – it's biological. Consider the children of Holocaust survivors. Studies show they carry biological markers of their parents' suffering, such as elevated stress hormones,[6] altered nervous system function, changes to brain structure[7] and increased susceptibility to anxiety and depression.[8] Similar patterns also appear in the descendants of enslaved peoples, Indigenous communities subjected to colonization, children raised in foster care, and families that endured war, famine, or forced displacement.[9]

Research suggests that trauma from three to five generations ago is carried through the RNA of the paternal line.[10] RNA (a molecule present in all living cells that's structurally similar to DNA) plays a key role in gene expression – passing on not just your genetic blueprint, but instructions for how that code is read and activated in response to the world around you.

To put this into perspective: In just 300 years, 11 generations of roughly 4,094 people contributed to your genetic makeup. That's 4,094 lives, decisions, hardships, and survival stories woven into your cells. The fact that we've only been able to study a handful of these generational impacts doesn't mean the rest don't exist, only that we haven't yet developed the tools to measure what many of us already intuitively know: We're carrying more than our own experience.

> *You're the living result of unbroken resilience. You're carrying stories of strength, bravery, and cellular memory of survival.*

You may also carry inherited survival strategies – behaviors and emotional patterns shaped not only by your ancestors' experiences but by the nervous systems of the caregivers who raised you. A mother who suppresses her emotions may teach her daughter, without ever saying a word, that feelings are unsafe. A family that lived through scarcity may unintentionally instill guilt around desire, rest, or abundance. These patterns aren't always spoken, but they are absorbed.

Healed Women Heal Generations

Trauma is stored in the body. But it's revealed in our relationships. And for women in marginalized communities, this inheritance is further layered by systemic forces that reach far beyond the family unit. Black women, Indigenous women, and women of color often carry not just personal trauma but also the accumulated physiological impact of racism, discrimination, and generational health inequities. The concept of 'racial weathering' explains how chronic exposure to these stressors compounds over time – leading to significantly higher rates of hypertension, autoimmune disease, and pregnancy complications.

Trans women, too – especially trans women of color – experience compounded trauma. Daily misgendering, social exclusion, gatekeeping in healthcare, and threats to physical safety all place an enormous burden on the nervous system, leading to disproportionate rates of anxiety, PTSD, and health disparities.

While this reality is neither fair nor just, lingering in that injustice without acting only deepens the wound. Anger is a valid and necessary response to oppression, but when it's left unprocessed or not transformed into meaningful action, it drains our vitality and keeps us tethered to the systems we're trying to transcend.

Healing ourselves, then, becomes a radical act of reclamation. It's not self-indulgence, but subversion; not merely personal, but profoundly collective and ancestral. By choosing to heal, we not only restore ourselves, we also participate in rewriting the story for those who came before us and those yet to come. This is exactly where our journey turns in the next chapter: from naming the wounds to rewiring our beliefs and patterns, and shaping a new legacy of liberation.

A Note About Blame

Before we move on, I want to speak directly to a misconception that often surfaces when I begin exploring trauma with my clients: that parents or caregivers are to blame for the later development of illness or symptoms in the children they raised.

This is not the message I'm sharing, and it's certainly not supported by any evidence. This work isn't about pointing fingers – it's about breaking patterns. Yes, our earliest environment shapes us, but all that means is that our parents or caregivers were shaped by theirs, too.

Love and trauma can coexist. If a parent's ability to express love is constrained, it's often because they, too, have experienced deep emotional pain. Most parents are simply doing the best they can with the resources, awareness, and capacity available to them at the time.

Just as children don't consciously choose their adaptive behaviors, parents don't either. Unless they've done the work to heal their own subconscious beliefs and regulate their nervous system, they'll pass down what they learned unconsciously and automatically. And while they're fully responsible for their children, they didn't create the world in which they must parent, either.

Take comfort in knowing that parental love is primal and infinite. It's hardwired into the brain. But love alone isn't always enough to protect a child from internalizing stress or adapting in ways that later become symptoms.

> *Pause for Self-Reflection*
>
> How do you currently view your childhood and those who shaped it? Respond to these questions in your journal:
>
> - *Is there a way to hold both your truth and others' limitations at the same time?*
> - *Can you feel the difference between blame and clarity?*
> - *Can you feel the difference between carrying pain and letting it move through you?*

If guilt, resistance, or defensiveness rises as you move through this work, take a breath. Let it move. You're here to interrupt a pattern and do it differently, not shame the ones who came before you.

Reframing Trauma

The more you understand trauma, the more you appreciate that your nervous system did what it had to do to keep you alive, connected, and protected in a world that didn't always feel safe. Gen Z has offered us a beautiful reframe for this: trauma as your origin story. Your hero's journey. Not in the sense that what happened was justified or deserved, but in that it shaped you as a protagonist. The one who survived. The one who gets to choose what comes next.

When you start to see your trauma this way – not as baggage but as the raw material from which your strength was forged – you stop trying to go back to who you were before. And you start becoming who you were always meant to be.

...

In the next chapter, we'll explore how your earliest environments and relationships wired your nervous system and subconscious mind for safety or survival, and take a crucial step toward reclaiming your authentic self-expression.

Chapter 12
REWIRING OUR WOUNDS

'The wound is where the light enters you.'

RUMI

I've lost count of the number of women who have come to me feeling exasperated because after years, sometimes decades, of talk therapy, they find themselves still trapped in the same patterns. They've unpacked their childhood trauma, dissected their triggers, and analyzed every relationship dynamic, yet their nervous system still reacts from a place of survival. They find themselves people-pleasing, overworking, jumping into fight mode, shutting down in conflict, binge eating, or feeling unsafe in moments that shouldn't logically warrant it.

This isn't because they're incapable of getting better. It's because trauma doesn't just live in the mind. It lives in the body. While traditional talk therapy is incredible for cultivating awareness, it has an average effectiveness rate of just 30 percent in resolving post-traumatic stress disorder (PTSD).[1]

That statistic suggests that when trauma is only approached cognitively with the conscious mind, we miss the very place where it's held: in the subconscious mind and nervous system. Often, talk therapy re-traumatizes the body by asking people to relive experiences of pain without giving them the proper physiological tools to process and release it. The following analogy explains why this is the case.

How Survival Gets Wired into the Body

Think of your inner world as a house equipped with a security system made up of the nervous system (the alarm), the subconscious mind (the alarm's control panel), the impact of trauma (which shapes the control panel's settings), and the conscious mind (the homeowner). Together, these components govern how you interpret, respond to, and protect yourself from perceived threats.

The Nervous System: the Alarm

Our nervous system constantly scans for danger – physical, emotional, or relational. When it's well regulated, it only sounds the alarm in true emergencies. But if it's been shaped by early trauma or chronic stress, it becomes oversensitive, setting off high-alert responses over minor cues such as facial expression, a change in tone, or a gut feeling.

The Subconscious Mind: the Alarm's Control Panel

Governing 90 percent of your thoughts, feelings, and behaviors, the subconscious determines what qualifies as danger based on past experiences and begins programming before you're even born, absorbing cues from your environment in utero.

As we discussed in Chapter 11, this programming deepens in your early childhood, especially during the first seven years, when your brain operates primarily in theta waves. If, during this time, you learned that anger leads to rejection or that love must be earned through perfection or compliance, your subconscious codes those experiences as threats. From then on, anything that even vaguely resembles those dynamics can trigger a survival response – because to your control panel, the past is always present.

Trauma: Shapes the Control Panel's Settings

Whether it's a big T trauma or a series of smaller, cumulative experiences that made you feel unseen, unsafe, or not enough (little t trauma), the subconscious stores them the same way, as evidence of danger. These moments don't have to be dramatic to leave an imprint – chronic invalidation, inconsistent caregiving, emotional neglect, or pressure to perform can all silently shape the control panel's settings.

Over time, your inner alarm begins to run on high-alert, interpreting everyday stressors – like a tone of voice, a delayed reply, or someone setting a boundary – as potential threats. This is why you might react intensely to situations that seem minor on the surface. Unless those subconscious beliefs are addressed and rewired, the alarm continues responding to the past, even when the present is safe.

The Conscious Mind: the Homeowner

As we discussed in Chapter 11, we don't fully move into our 'house' until our mid-twenties – when our brain finishes maturing. By that point, the nervous system (alarm) and the subconscious mind (control panel) have been running on autopilot for years, shaping our reactions without our awareness. We might logically understand that we're safe now, but our body doesn't get the memo. It's still responding based on outdated programming.

Of course, the rewiring of our subconscious can begin long before our twenties (and at any age) – but without the level of conscious awareness that typically develops in our mid-twenties, we're more likely to keep living out patterns we never consciously chose.

The Survival Loop

I hope this analogy enables you to see why so many of the emotional, behavioral, and relational patterns addressed by the Root Restoration Framework (see Chapter 8) can feel so automatic, sticky, and difficult to shift.

You may have noticed the way one unexpected text can send your heart racing, or a subtle shift in someone's tone makes you instantly backtrack on your boundaries. These aren't overreactions. They're survival strategies. And when those strategies have been reinforced for years, it can feel like you're going round in circles rather than forward. This trauma response cycle is what I call the survival loop.

You may already feel like you're caught in the survival loop – triggered by the same kind of stressor, reaching for the same coping strategy, and then wondering why you can't seem to change. That's because until you work at the level of the nervous system and the subconscious mind – the level where the original programming lives – your system will keep looping back to what it knows.

As James Hollis, a Jungian psychoanalyst explains in his book *Finding Meaning in the Second Half of Life*, 'No one awakens in the morning, looks in the mirror, and says, "I think I will repeat my mistakes today." But, frequently, this replication of history is precisely what we do, because we are unaware of the silent presence of those programmed energies, the core ideas we've acquired, internalized, and surrendered to.

Let's look more closely at how the survival loop is activated, and then I'll explain how we can interrupt it.

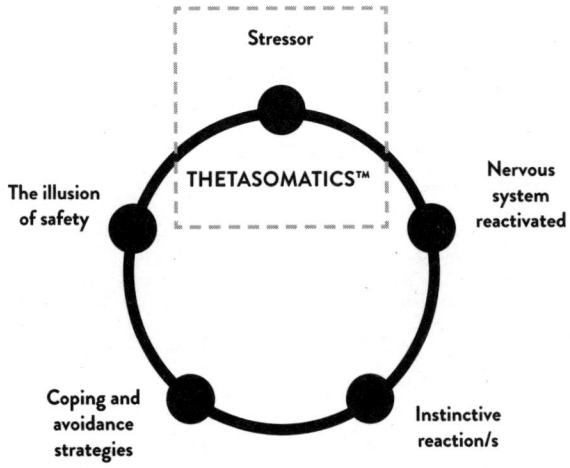

The survival loop

Here's an overview of the stages of the loop.

Stressor (Trigger)

The loop begins when something in your environment – a tone, a facial expression, a delay or reaction – triggers a response that your subconscious has previously associated with danger. It doesn't matter whether the current event is big or small. What matters is what it reminds your nervous system of.

This is where trauma lives: in the stored association, not the situation itself. Trauma isn't just the memory of what happened – it's how your body learned to protect you in response. So, when a present-day event resembles something painful or unsafe from your past, your system responds as if it's happening all over again. Here are some examples:

- A friend cancels plans at the last minute – *triggers* the subconscious belief: 'Something about me must be too much or not enough.'

- A partner expresses mild frustration with us – *triggers* the subconscious belief: 'If someone is upset with me, I'm at risk of being abandoned.'

In both cases, the current experience lights up an old wound. The stressor is real, but it's the meaning beneath it, stored in your subconscious and nervous system, that activates the survival loop.

Nervous System Reactivated

At this stage, your body responds as if the original trauma is happening again; not to the situation itself, but to what it reminds you of.

Instinctive Reaction(s)

The nervous system then chooses the reaction(s) that once helped you survive (fight-flight/freeze or fawn). This can look like people-pleasing to avoid conflict, shutting down to prevent escalation, or over-controlling to feel safe. Even if it no longer serves you, your body repeats what it knows.

Coping and Avoidance Strategies

When your nervous system is activated, you instinctively reach for something to regulate it. Most of us were never taught how to return to the parasympathetic nervous system in healthy ways, so we turn to numbing strategies we've seen modelled such as scrolling on our phone, drinking, binge eating, overexercising, or overworking. In contrast, healthy regulating strategies look like breathwork, movement, journaling, music, laughter, hugs with a safe person or grounding in nature.

The Illusion of Safety

These coping and avoidance strategies create the illusion of safety and control, but because they don't address the underlying beliefs in the subconscious, the nervous system will continue perceiving the stressor you've reacted to as a threat in the future.

For example, if a difficult conversation made your body feel unsafe, doing 10 minutes of breathwork might soothe the activation this time, but if the deeper belief is 'It's not safe for me to share my needs,' the same trigger will activate you once more, moving you back through the survival loop all over again.

> *Pause for Self-Reflection*
>
> Think about or journal on the following questions:
>
> - *Is there a pattern or reaction you keep finding yourself in, even when you 'know better'?*
> - *What might this loop be protecting you from feeling, remembering, or risking?*
> - *What would safety look like in that moment instead?*

Let's look at two examples of how the survival loop can play out in real-life situations:

Olivia and Samantha's Stories

Olivia was reading a passage from a textbook out loud to the class in elementary school biology when she accidentally pronounced the word 'organism' as 'orgasm.' (The kind of verbal slip that so many of us have made.) Her classmates erupted with laughter, and for years afterward, they continued to tease her, calling her 'Orgasm Olivia' and making up songs and sounds to mock her.

Even as the joke's origin was lost to time, the nickname lingered among Olivia's male peers, embedding itself into her sense of self in ways they never saw. This experience lodged two key beliefs in her subconscious mind: 'My voice leads to humiliation' and 'I need to express myself perfectly or I'll experience shame.'

Decades later, these thought loops were holding her back as she took on more responsibility as a director in a marketing firm. She struggled to sleep before big client presentations and found herself getting extremely anxious, sweating and angrily snapping at her team. Her nervous system was interpreting the upcoming presentation as a threat based on her childhood experience, and to cope, she'd mindlessly snack on potato chips until she returned to a state of calm.

Meanwhile, Samantha grew up in a household where love was only verbally or physically expressed when she achieved something – being a straight-A student, excelling in sports, or winning an essay competition. If she failed, she felt invisible. Her subconscious learned: 'You're only lovable when you're perfect.'

Today, as a small-business owner also juggling motherhood, she finds it nearly impossible to rest without feeling guilty. Whenever she tries to slow down, a familiar sense of panic creeps in. To feel in control, she overworks, over-delivers, and takes on more than she can handle. Her body is exhausted, but rest feels unsafe. When she does attempt to relax, she numbs out by binge-watching TV shows or making endless to-do lists for the following day.

Interrupting the Survival Loop

My therapeutic method ThetaSomatics™ is designed to interrupt the survival loop at its source. It cultivates safety and resilience in mind (*theta*) and body (*somatics*) by rewiring the nervous system and the subconscious adaptive beliefs we've picked up throughout our lives. Rather than trying to think your way out of old behaviors or simply talk through your pain, this approach works at the level where the beliefs that drive them were first wired in.

In Chapter 21, I'll guide you through a ThetaSomatics™ Rewiring Practice (*see pages 241–48*). But right now, let's see why this and other somatic healing techniques are such powerful tools for rewiring trauma and subconscious wounds.

The Subconscious Mind (Theta State)

The subconscious mind operates 90 percent of the time, storing the beliefs, fears, and patterns that guide your daily life. The most direct way to access and rewire it is through theta, a naturally occurring brainwave state that we enter as we fall asleep, wake up, meditate, engage in breathwork, or drop into a trance or hypnosis.

In the theta state, the subconscious becomes highly suggestible. This is where old neural pathways such as 'I'm not lovable' can be gently replaced with new neural pathways such as 'I'm lovable just as I am' or 'I'm worthy of unconditional love.' This process is made possible by neuroplasticity – the brain's remarkable ability to change its structure and function.

These neural pathways then shape the way your nervous system responds to future stressors. Instead of defaulting to stress, anxiety, or panic (fight-or-flight activation), you begin to access perspective, calm, and clarity because your system has learned a new way to interpret, relate, and respond to the event (stressor), as shown in this diagram:

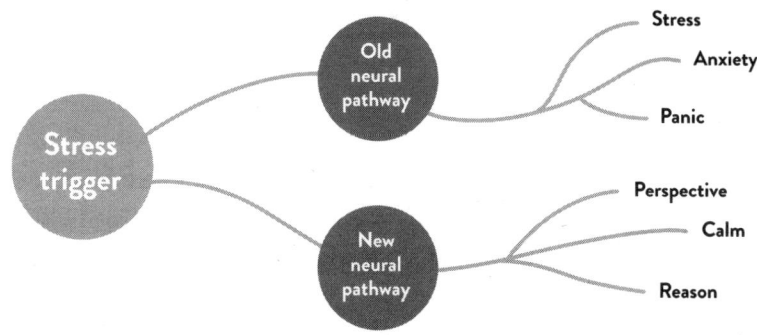

The process of neuroplasticity

Through nervous system regulation, guided visualization, inner dialogue, intentional affirmations, and neuroplasticity-enhancing activities such as dance, the ThetaSomatics™ Rewiring Practice (*see pages 241–48*) helps you form new neural pathways in the brain – rewiring your felt experience of the world over time.

The Nervous System (Somatic Healing)

The nervous system is responsible for 80 percent of your body's signals. By discharging stored tension or emotions and restoring a sense of internal safety, somatic healing work moves you from reactivity to regulation.

Practices such as rocking, tremoring, shaking, dance, and character work recalibrate the body's baseline, so that what once felt overwhelming becomes tolerable; you'll learn how to use these tools in Chapters 20 and 21. Over time, you'll not just react differently, you'll cultivate an inner sense of safety which signals to your body that it's time to shift its focus and resources to healing and self-repair.

This process is made possible by bioplasticity, the body's innate ability to reshape itself based on input, environment, and experience. It's happening inside you all the time. For example, your skin renews itself every 28 days, your stomach lining regenerates every few days, and your bones, though solid, remodel continuously.

Your Triggers Are Clues

Your nervous system will always choose a familiar hell over an unfamiliar heaven. This is why a chaotic relationship may unconsciously feel more 'normal' to you than a calm one – not because it's better but because your body knows how to survive it. Left unhealed, the nervous system will always guide you back to what it knows, even if what it knows is pain.

We've been taught to fear discomfort, to interpret our triggers as signs that something's wrong with us. But in fact, those triggers are proof that something's unfinished. They highlight the areas where outdated survival patterns are quietly dictating our reactions. Instead of running from these moments, ThetaSomatics invites you to treat your patterns (whether they are people-pleasing, overworking, or numbing) as clues.

As the relationship therapist Vienna Pharaon so wisely puts it in her book *The Origins of You*: 'Avoiding your triggers isn't healing. Healing happens when you're triggered and you're able to move through the pain, the pattern, and the story and walk your way to a different ending.'

Each reaction and behavioral pattern is a doorway to deeper understanding, an invitation to reclaim the parts of you that have been sidelined for the sake of safety. The more we rewrite our beliefs on a subconscious and nervous system level, the more we embody our full, unapologetic selves. Here's a story that shows what becomes possible when you stop reacting from your wound and begin responding from your worth.

Amelia's Story

Amelia, a 28-year-old from the Netherlands, had been trying to conceive for three years. She and her partner had tracked ovulation with military precision, overhauled their diets, taken supplements, and endured the monthly roller-coaster of hope and heartbreak. All tests came back normal, and the doctors called it unexplained infertility. But deep down, Amelia knew there was more to it.

When she arrived in my world, she was exhausted – physically, emotionally, and spiritually. In our first session, I asked her gently, 'If your body was protecting you from something by not falling pregnant, what might that be?' She blinked at me, confused. Then her eyes filled with tears.

Amelia had grown up in a household where motherhood looked like martyrdom. Her own mother had suffered deeply – sacrificing her dreams, losing her sense of self in endless caregiving, and slowly becoming bitter and withdrawn. As a child, Amelia absorbed the subconscious belief that to be a good mother, she had to put herself last. That being a mother meant being exhausted, selfless to the point of invisibility, and always running on empty.

She'd spent her adult life living the opposite way – traveling, building a career, cultivating freedom and self-expression. And although she longed for a child, her subconscious was running on a program of fear, repeating Pregnancy equals sacrifice. Motherhood equals loss of self.

So, together, we began to gently rewrite the story. We used somatic work to regulate her nervous system, hypnosis in the theta state to meet the inner child still bracing against becoming her mother, and ThetaSomatics to install new beliefs: 'I can be a mother and still be myself. I can create new life without losing mine.' Amelia created a new normal for herself by only consuming social media posts from women who embodied these beliefs – consistently giving her subconscious proof that living this way was possible.

Amelia also started reconnecting to joy, pleasure, and creativity to reclaim safety in her body. She let go of timelines. She softened. And three months later, she conceived naturally. It wasn't magic: It was biology, energy, and belief, finally aligned. When the body no longer perceived motherhood as a threat, it allowed it in.

At the core of this work is an unshakable truth: *It's safe to be who you are and live life on your own terms.* In fact, the world *needs* you to be who you are. Because real solutions to today's crises – whether personal, social, or global – won't come from conformity or compliance. They'll come from the diverse, vibrant voices of those who have reclaimed their power from the forces that sought to suppress them.

...

Now that you understand how survival gets wired into your body, it's time to explore a force that keeps you playing small: shame. In the next chapter, we'll break down how shame shapes what's known as the adaptive self, why it's been used to control women for centuries, and how reclaiming your authenticity is the first act of true rebellion.

Chapter 13

THE ADAPTIVE SELF VS. THE AUTHENTIC SELF

'Illness not only has a history, but it tells a history. It is a culmination of a lifelong history of struggle for self.'

GABOR MATÉ

Shame. Shame. Shame. If you've watched the TV show *Game of Thrones*, you'll likely remember the infamous Walk of Shame scene from Season 5. Cersei Lannister – regal, ruthless, and once the most powerful woman in the land of Westeros – is dragged from her gilded castle and forced to walk naked through the filthy streets of King's Landing. Her long, golden hair is hacked short, her body exposed to the sneers and jeers of a merciless crowd, who spit on her, pelt her with rotten food, and scream insults. And a Septa (female clergy of the dominant religion) rings a bell with cruel precision, chanting *shame* with each clang.

Cersei's power isn't taken by force but dismantled through exposure, degradation, and psychological warfare. It's a vivid fictional depiction of how patriarchal systems, under the guise of religious morality, have long weaponized shame to control women's bodies and identities. By transforming female transgression into public entertainment, it mirrors the deep entanglement of religion, patriarchy, and capitalism.

Most of us will never be paraded naked through the streets as punishment, but the architecture of shame – the threats of humiliation, the omnipresent gaze of judgment, the systemic stripping-away of dignity – remains firmly in place. Whether through online harassment, cancel culture, or the more insidious everyday shaming women endure for the way we look, love, live, and lead, the message is consistent: *conform, or be exposed.*

In a world where the currency of shame flows through media headlines, social feeds, and cultural narratives, it's become society's sharpest tool of control. Wielded against women to remind them of the cost of stepping out of line.

Shame: A Cultural Weapon

Shame is a key shaper of the adaptive self – the version of you that prioritizes safety over authenticity and compliance over courage. It's the voice in your head that tells you to stay small, keep quiet, dim your light, convincing you that doing so is the only way to survive.

Instead of playing to win, you begin playing it safe. It's why you hesitate to apply for that promotion, why you shrink around people who intimidate you, why you feel like an imposter in rooms in which you've *earned* your place. But, as the two previous chapters have shown, the adaptive self is a survival strategy crafted within a culture that rewards women for their compliance and punishes them for their audacity.

> *We learn to adapt because the systems around us demand it. And while our adaptive self may feel like protection, it's a prison disguised as safety.*

The painful emotion of shame evolved to serve a productive purpose. In the harsh conditions of early human life, shame ensured cooperation, nudging us to align with group norms to secure connection, belonging, and the communal care essential for survival, particularly for women tasked with nurturing the next generation.

It was meant to be a temporary corrective, not a permanent state. Yet of course, that's exactly what happened. As human societies became more complex, hierarchical and patriarchal shame morphed into a mechanism of enforcing conformity, particularly around gender roles. For women, shame became the invisible leash, used to police our bodies, desires, and ambitions under the guise of morality, tradition, or even love. Religion institutionalized shame, capitalism commodified it, and patriarchy embedded it into cultural narratives so that it now feels like second nature.

Why Women Police Other Women

When men are shamed, it's usually for what they *do* – failure, weakness, or breaking the rules. But when women are shamed, it's for *who we are*. When a woman is assaulted, mistreated, or violated, the first question society asks isn't what happened to her but what did she do to deserve it? The blame lands squarely on her shoulders: was it her clothes, her choices, her inability to 'see the signs'? This conditioning starts early, teaching women that when harm is done to us, the shame is ours to carry. And we've internalized this message so deeply that it's become self-perpetuating. Shame is such a painful learning experience that we've learned to wield it not only against ourselves but against each other, reinforcing the systems that keep us small.

When a woman dares to step outside the boundaries of what's deemed 'acceptable' – whether she's too loud, too ambitious, too sexual, or too assertive – it's often other women who are quickest to criticize. We judge both the new mother who returns to work 'too soon' *and* the one who stays at home. We whisper about the woman who embraces her sexuality, calling her 'attention-seeking,' while praising another for being 'modest.'

But this isn't because women are inherently judgmental. It's because we've been taught that the safest way to survive in a system designed to shame us is to align ourselves with it. By pointing the finger at other women, we attempt to deflect attention from ourselves. We create distance from behaviors society punishes, believing (often unconsciously) that if we conform and uphold these unspoken rules, we'll secure safety for ourselves.

The Language of Shame

To truly emancipate ourselves, we must stop indulging in shaming and, instead, support one another in living authentically. We must cheer on other women for being loud, ambitious, sensual, and assertive so we begin to dismantle the systems that rely on our silence, our compliance, and our complicity. To do that, we must recognize the ways that shame has been woven into our daily lives and internal filters

From the moment we enter the world, we're handed an invisible rulebook. Some of it is spoken. Most of it is not. In my childhood home, the rules were explicit. There was a piece of paper taped to the kitchen counter, color-coded like a traffic light: Do what you have to do (green). Then, do what you should do (orange). Lastly, do what you want to do (red).

I lived by these rules. Green first: obligations, responsibilities, non-negotiables. Then orange: the tasks that make you a good person, daughter, older sister, and student. And finally, if there was any time or energy left over, red: what you actually want. The fun. The freedom. The joy. The creativity. But the color-coding told the real story: What I *wanted* was wrong. Selfish. Shameful.

My parents are thoughtful people who raised their children with care and intention. I'm sure their only aim was to instill simple routines such as finish your homework before playing outside and brush your teeth before bed. But for me, these rules reinforced a deeper lesson I was already internalizing through school, society, and culture – that my desires were secondary. Being 'good' wasn't about who I was; it was about how useful I could be.

Even now, I still catch myself in the grip of a 'should,' but thankfully my partner gently reflects back to me the subtle self-betrayal hidden in that word. Because 'should' is the language of shame. It punishes the past version of you for not knowing what you now know. It's an insidious form of internalized aggression that keeps us and our nervous systems on edge – bracing, contracted, and armoring for protection.

> *Pause for Self-Reflection*
>
> Consider where these messages we've explored about shame, self-sacrifice, and conformity have seeped into your own life.
>
> - *Where have you instinctively placed obligation before joy?*
> - *Where have you been conditioned to believe that being 'good' means being 'selfless'?*
> - *Where have you muted your own needs – shrinking, softening, silencing – to maintain harmony, to keep the peace, to avoid being labelled as 'too much'?*

Now picture a woman who refuses to play by these rules. A woman who moves through the world unapologetically. She prioritizes her needs without hesitation, says 'no' without explanation, and claims her desires without shrinking to make others comfortable. She speaks her mind freely, expressing the full spectrum of her emotions – anger, joy, sadness, pleasure – without shame or self-consciousness.

What words come to mind when you see her? Obnoxious? Selfish? Bitch? Difficult? Entitled? Crazy? Now imagine a man with the same traits. What do you call him? Powerful? A leader? Ambitious?

Stepping into Our Authentic Self

This is the insidious double bind of femininity. The cycle of self-abandonment doesn't always begin with overt abuse or dramatic neglect; more often, it's forged in the small, repeated moments when a girl learns that her authentic self-expression is inconvenient, too loud, too needy, too emotional. Over time, she internalizes the message that her true self is unacceptable – or worse, unlovable. But what we once learned for safety, we can now unlearn for healing. Just because it's imprinted, doesn't mean it's permanent.

So, when the urge to shrink arises, pause. Take a breath, and ask yourself: *Is this truly me? Or is this who I was told I had to be to be loved?* Healing begins in the small, everyday moments where you choose yourself. Over and over again. This is how shame loses its hold on you. Not all at once, but choice by choice, until your truth feels safer than your programming.

> *Each time you honor your needs instead of overriding them, or speak your truth instead of swallowing it, you're laying a new foundation rooted in self-worth, not shame.*

For women, authenticity is a radical act. It's a luxury – a privilege afforded to those who have either escaped or unlearned the socialization that demands us to be palatable, agreeable, and self-sacrificing. The cost of stepping into our full selves remains perilously high. Speaking your truth can still cost you relationships. Setting boundaries can cost you approval. Prioritizing your needs can cost you belonging. And in a society that equates belonging with survival, that risk feels life-threatening.

Now, if you're feeling the weight of roles that you never consciously chose, or if you've spent years contorting yourself to fit expectations that were never truly your own, then know this: your authenticity is not lost. It's simply been buried, layered beneath years of conditioning, survival strategies, and patterns inherited from generations of women who were taught the same lessons.

That version of you – the one who is whole, vibrant, unapologetic – is still there. We'll talk a lot more about reconnecting with our authentic self in Chapter 17.

Reclaiming Our Voice

My favorite Disney film is *The Little Mermaid*. As a child, I felt an unspoken connection to the protagonist, Ariel, because, like her, I knew what it felt like to lose my voice. Ariel literally trades her voice for the chance to belong, to be loved, to step into the life she dreams of. And in many ways, this mirrors the unspoken contract women are taught to accept: Sacrifice your voice, your truth, your unfiltered self-expression in exchange for acceptance and safety.

The scene that haunted me is where Ariel reclaims her voice from the sea witch, Ursula, who embodies everything manipulative and oppressive about power. Ursula is master of exploitation, preying on Ariel's insecurities and desires. She had convinced Ariel that losing her voice – her most powerful asset – was the price of being loved.

In reclaiming her voice, Ariel doesn't just recover something she'd lost; she also *owns* her power and her ability to shape her own destiny. This idea planted seeds of recognition deep within me: Our voice isn't just a tool for communication – it's the very essence of who we are.

So, when *The Little Mermaid* was reimagined with Black actress Halle Bailey as Ariel, I was elated. Watching a story that had shaped my childhood expand to reflect a broader, richer reality was more than just a win for representation, it was a cultural correction.

It sent a message to every little girl, especially those who historically have been omitted from these narratives: *Your voice matters. Your story belongs.* Encouraging them to stay connected to their authentic self-expression as an act of defiance against every system that's told them to quiet down, stay small, and make themselves palatable.

Our Power Pipeline: The Womb-Throat Axis

As I grew older and began to understand the body's innate intelligence, I realized that 'finding your voice' isn't merely a metaphor – it's a physiological necessity. Studies have connected self-silencing to conditions including irritable bowel syndrome, HIV, chronic fatigue syndrome, and cancer among women.[1]

But beyond these alarming links, there's an even more profound layer – one that touches the very core of who we are. Our voice is the wellspring of our creativity and the conduit of our self-expression. It turns out that our ability to speak new life in the form of ideas and words as well as create new human life are deeply connected.

Women are biologically and energetically designed to be creators, leaders, and truth-tellers. And our voice and our womb are intricately linked through what I call the 'power pipeline,' a sacred axis which, when fully activated, transforms not just individual lives but the world at large. The tissues, structures, and organs in the womb–throat axis – the vocal cords, vulva, larynx, womb, and pelvic floor – have striking visual and schematic similarities, as the illustration below shows.

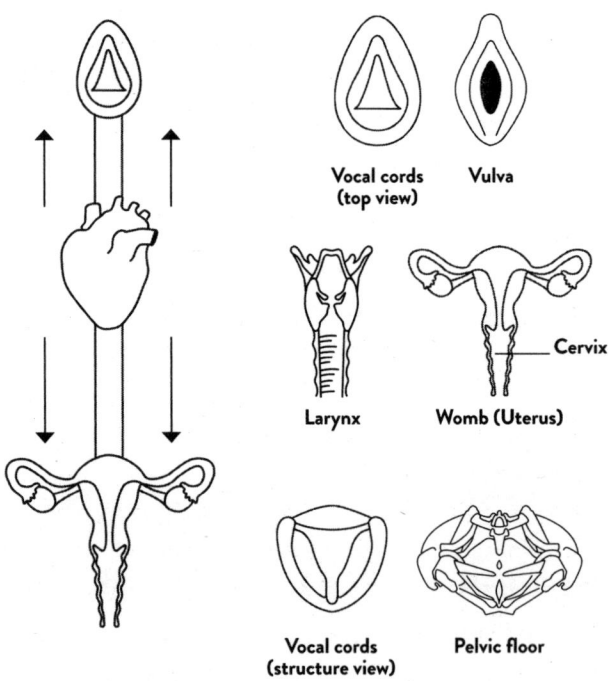

Structures in the womb–throat axis

They also have profound biological connections. Let's dive into these and also look at ways you can activate your power pipeline. We'll also explore the central role played by the heart.

Vocal Cords and Vulva

The vocal cords and the vulva are gateways of expression and release. They both open and close in response to internal cues of safety, desire, or danger. When a woman feels unsafe, both areas instinctively contract (which is why sex can feel uncomfortable when she's not fully relaxed). When she feels secure, seen, and sovereign, they soften and open.

The labia (the folds of skin that form part of the vulva) and vocal cords are both finely attuned to emotion. Think of how your voice shakes when you're about to cry or how numb the vulva can feel after betrayal or sexual trauma.

Pipeline Activation: Vocal silence and vulval disconnection often coexist. Voice reclamation and sexual healing are therefore intertwined, and healing one often begins to unlock the other. This is your nudge to begin voicing your desires in the bedroom (and every area of your life) if this is something you struggle with!

Larynx and Womb

From an embryological perspective, the larynx and cervix (the lower portion of the womb) develop from the same tissue, which is why, during labor, relaxing the jaw and releasing low, open sounds can help the cervix soften and dilate. Midwives have long said: 'A tight jaw equals a tight cervix.'

Both the larynx and the womb are cyclical, expressive, and hormonally responsive. They open and close, swell and contract, according to our inner state. When one is constricted, the other often follows. When one is liberated, the other softens too.

The womb responds to stress, fear, grief, and trauma through subtle contractions, storing unresolved emotional tension within its fascia (the connective tissue that surrounds and supports muscles, organs, and nerves). This is why the womb is often referred to as a second heart – it doesn't just hold life; it holds memory.

Pipeline Activation: Your womb may be carrying echoes of the women who came before you: their silence, their suppression, their fight to belong. When you release what's stored there by using your voice, you don't just heal yourself, you heal your lineage. The hip-opening and sound-activation exercises you'll be guided through in Chapter 20 (*see pages 221–23*) are designed to help facilitate this release.

Vocal Cords and Pelvic Floor

These structures are connected through fascia, meaning tension in the throat often echoes in the pelvic floor, and vice versa. This is why trauma stored in the pelvic floor can manifest as vocal constriction, while breathwork or vocal expression can initiate release below.

Pipeline Activation: Try the hip-opening and sound-activation exercises in Chapter 20.

Open Your Heart

The vagus nerve – the body's main regulator of the parasympathetic nervous system – flows through the vocal cords, heart, lungs, diaphragm, digestive organs, all the way down to your womb, creating a visceral thread that connects your ability to express, feel, and create.

At the center of your power pipeline, therefore, is your heart. Not just anatomically but energetically. It's the gateway between your womb and your voice. The filter that determines how – if at all – your inner desires get expressed in the external world.

And its power isn't just symbolic. The heart generates an electrical field that's approximately 60 times stronger than the brain and an electromagnetic field that's thousands of times greater (one that can be measured several feet away from the body).

So, when your heart is guarded or closed, the signals moving between your womb and throat become scrambled. You may speak from fear instead of truth. You may create from obligation instead of inspiration. But when your heart is open, it becomes the portal of coherence. An open heart sends clear signals of safety both down to the womb and up to the voice. Bringing your brain, breath, and blood pressure into the optimal state for healing.[2]

Returning to Our Full Expression

Living with an open heart is true feminine power. And it's something I had to relearn. Growing up, I wasn't always Isabella. I was Issy. Then Izzy. And eventually, Izzi. Each iteration of my name throughout my adolescence was a survival strategy to be palatable, productive, armored, and protected.

The shortening of my name mirrored the closing of my heart. I thought strength meant being impenetrable. But real strength is the ability to stay soft, open, heart-centered, and emotionally honest without losing your boundaries. Reclaiming my full name in my twenties was a huge moment for me. It was a return to femininity and my full expression. To softness as strength. To taking up emotional and vocal space.

And this isn't just my story – it's the unspoken inheritance of most women. We live in a world that rewards head-over-heart logic and punishes heart-led presence. A world that glorifies productivity and dismisses intuition. Here's a story that illustrates this.

Georgina's Story

Georgina Capdevila was born and raised in Catalonia, Spain – a land rich in cultural heritage yet scarred by a past in which speaking the local language, Catalan, and singing its songs was forbidden as recently as 50 years ago under the dictatorship of Francisco Franco. 'Most of my ancestors were from Catalonia,' Georgina told me when we met on a retreat, making it very clear she felt the epigenetic markers of that trauma.

Georgina's instinct to repress her authentic voice was compounded throughout her childhood years while studying music, where her natural singing voice was reshaped by strict standards. 'I felt I had to hit the right note every time, or else I wasn't good enough,' she explained, describing how the pressure to perform perfectly – singing from her head and playing the flute for precision rather than from her heart for genuine expression – eventually eroded her ability to express herself unfiltered, even in daily life.

In her twenties, Georgina moved to London and began working for the University of the Arts – a prestigious role that nevertheless left her profoundly unfulfilled. 'Deep down, I was running away from my home and my past,' she admitted. As she tried to escape, her body began to signal distress: painful periods, persistent pain throughout her cycle, and an unexplained discharge that left doctors baffled.

Initially, Georgina put up with the mounting lack of answers. But then, in a moment of vulnerability, she summoned the courage to use her voice for the first time in years: to demand fidelity from her romantic partner. 'He broke his promise, and even called to tell me he had chlamydia,' she recalled. Although her STI test came back negative, the deep pain of that betrayal marked a decisive turning point. 'I realized I wasn't loving myself enough or listening to my body's signs,' she confided.

Determined to finally understand what her body was trying to tell her, Georgina found a gynecologist, who suggested she was suffering with PCOS, although all her tests came back 'normal.' At the same time, she began exploring spirituality – diving into tarot, astrology, and eventually, a womb-healing course, which offered her far more clarity than doctors appointments. 'When your womb awakens, your voice awakens,' she reflected. In a breakthrough moment, she was finally able to tell her mother she loved her, following decades of emotional repression and distance between them. A sentiment her mother then echoed to her own mother, breaking a cycle of silence across three generations.

Georgina's journey continued when she met and married a much older man, and together they began hosting sound-healing sessions where

Georgina spontaneously started singing again. Her voice, once silenced by perfectionism, emerged as a potent medicine for those who attended.

While at the time she thought she'd entered the conscious partnership she'd been dreaming of, she says, 'there was still a thick veil I wasn't seeing.' It wasn't until 2023 that her best friend reflected a hard truth: Georgina wasn't truly attracted to her husband. She confessed that she'd nearly run away from her wedding the day before but stayed, paralyzed by the fear of using her voice and trusting her inner knowing. That insight – made possible through loving sisterhood – led to her divorce, and once she finally left that relationship, her symptoms vanished.

Finally, in 2024, Georgina's subconscious surfaced a memory in an Ayahuasca ceremony that connected all the pieces of the puzzle – childhood sexual abuse by a much older man. This trauma explained her decision to marry someone so senior despite her deep reservations. 'The nervous system seeks what's normal and what it knows – I wanted to change at the time, but I couldn't,' she reflected. 'Now, whenever I doubt myself, I always remember that I was able to tell my family the truth about my abuse, and that gives me courage. I know that the worst is behind me, and I can do or say anything.'

Now 32, symptom- and PCOS-free, Georgina has channeled her own transformative journey into empowering other women to reclaim their voices and follow their heart's desire through her work as a Voice Alchemist Mentor. I asked her, 'In your view, what does a woman who has reclaimed her voice look like?' She smiled, closed her eyes, and spoke from her heart: 'A woman who isn't afraid to shine her light – to be her most expressive self, without worrying about how her past or present lands on others. She trusts herself, focuses solely on being herself and expressing what is in her heart. She praises other women and celebrates herself.'

I then asked, 'What does a world look like where every woman reclaims her voice?' And her answer came out like a song, a tender, lilting melody: 'Each of us has a voice – a unique instrument in a cosmic orchestra. We don't compare our flute with someone else's piano – we all express ourselves in *different, beautiful ways. We each trust our intuition and trust our channel. And together we'll create a symphony of healing and transformation across generations. Our whole ecosystem will function as it should.'*

Breaking Free of Obedience

There's a widespread belief in high-performance culture that feminine qualities such as empathy and emotional depth are liabilities. But feminine, heart-centered power isn't frivolous. It's not a distraction from what matters. It *is* what matters.

Because of women's ability to create new life and our parallels with nature, we're always connected to something greater than ourselves. That's why our desires feel wild, creative, even unreasonable to the masculine. We don't just dream big – we see a future where everyone is nourished, healthy, and joyful. We know that future is possible, and that it's not a delusion. Your heart's desires aren't selfish or indulgent. They're a signal. A call from your womb to bring something new into form.

> *Owning your feminine power means reclaiming your right to desire, to dream, and to channel those dreams through your heart and voice into reality.*

When women are in their power, they want more. They feel more. They create more. They take up more space. And in a world that doesn't reflect back that it's safe to do that, it's easy to internalize lack: *If I desire it and it doesn't exist (or someone tells me I can't), maybe I'm too much. Maybe I'm not enough.*

But the powerful feminine doesn't fall for that lie. She knows: *If I desire it, it's because I'm meant to create it.* This shift – owning your authentic wants, needs, and dreams – is radical. It redefines success and refuses to outsource authority and ability.

The world doesn't need more women following the rules. It needs women who rewrite them. Women who birth new models – ones that prioritize intuition over control, creativity over conformity, and collaboration over competition. But to *voice* those desires and actively pursue them requires something we've been taught to fear: facing and reclaiming the full spectrum of our emotional truth. And no emotion has been more systematically silenced, more culturally vilified, or more deeply feared than anger.

Angry Women

Anger isn't just an emotion, it's a biological signal hardwired into our brain through the rage system, designed to protect our boundaries and assert our needs. It's the instinctual *no* – the immediate, visceral pushback when our integrity is threatened.

But for women, this natural response has been recast as something dangerous, unruly, and shameful. From an early age, we're taught to suppress our anger, to swap it out for politeness, compliance, and emotional labor. While anger repression isn't exclusive to women, it's imposed on us more pervasively, with far-reaching consequences that echo through our minds, bodies, and relationships.

Even women at the pinnacle of power aren't spared. In her deeply self-aware memoir *Becoming*, former First Lady Michelle Obama reflects on how meticulously she had to manage perceptions of her assertiveness to avoid being labelled as 'angry' or 'intimidating.' The stereotype of the 'angry Black woman' became a weapon, wielded to undermine her authority and diminish her voice.

Obama's experience reflects a broader cultural narrative: Women who express anger risk punishment, while those who remain compliant and emotionally restrained are rewarded. Women are conditioned to shoulder discomfort silently and to swallow, or suppress, their rage to maintain the illusion of harmony.

The Cost of Self-Silencing

But there's a crucial difference between *suppression* and *repression*. Suppression is conscious – you *know* you're biting your tongue. Repression, however, buries anger so deeply you don't even realize it's there. It festers beneath the surface, emerging not as righteous indignation but as unexplained tears, compulsive eating, or relentless busyness.

This chronic repression leads to self-silencing – the habitual erasure of our thoughts, feelings, and needs to avoid conflict and maintain relationships, particularly intimate ones. We've been programmed to be nice, to smooth things over, to keep the peace at all costs.

The effects of burying our anger are staggering. In March 2022 a team of researchers at the University of Pittsburgh in the US discovered that women of color who strongly agreed with statements like 'I rarely express my anger to those close to me' were 70 percent more likely to experience increased carotid atherosclerosis, a cardiovascular plaque associated with higher risk of heart attack.[3]

Anger, when expressed constructively, is a life-affirming force. But when buried, it metastasizes – transforming into anxiety, depression, chronic illness, and even premature death.

> ### *Pause for Self-Reflection*
>
> Before you move on, think about or journal on the following:
>
> - *What messages did I receive growing up about expressing anger, especially as a woman?*
> - *How do I currently respond when anger arises in me? Is there a boundary I've ignored or a truth I've swallowed in order to stay 'safe' or liked?*
> - *What might become possible if I let myself feel and express my anger with power and purpose?*

I recently had a powerful conversation over brunch with my friend Tamu Thomas, a Black British woman who's dedicated nearly two decades of her career to social work and written the wonderful book *Women Who Work Too Much*. As we discussed expressing healthy anger, she shared something so poetic I had to pull out my notebook and write it down: 'When a fire burns, the ash fertilizes the soil and spurs new growth – the same is true for our anger.'

This insight captures precisely why society fears women's anger. When a woman reconnects with this powerful emotion, she also reconnects with her boundaries, her worth, and her inherent strength. Women who reclaim their rage don't just transform themselves – they ignite revolutions and reshape systems.

Express, Don't Explain, Yourself

For a woman, naming your desires and voicing your needs without justification is an act of rebellion. Absurd, isn't it? That authenticity, the simple audacity to exist in the fullness of who you are, is still revolutionary in a world that profits from our silence.

In a study tracking nearly 4,000 people in Framingham, Massachusetts, over a decade, researchers found that women who swallowed their emotions during marital conflicts were four times more likely to die prematurely than those who spoke up.[4] *Four times.* That's an epidemic of self-abandonment, normalized by a culture that praises women for being agreeable, adaptable, and endlessly accommodating.

> *From the 'chill' girlfriend to the selfless mother,*
> *womanhood is shaped by the myth that our*
> *highest virtue is knowing how to disappear.*

We're trained to contort, to comply, to make ourselves smaller in service of harmony. But what's harmonious about a body at war with itself? What's noble about burying your truth so deeply it begins to fester beneath your skin?

The women I work with always echo similar refrains: 'I don't deserve to put my needs first – I'm not the breadwinner.' Or the classic, 'I don't want to be selfish' or 'I said yes, again, even though every part of me screamed no.' These daily acts of self-betrayal accumulate like sediment in the body until they harden into illness, infertility, fatigue, or chronic pain. In trying to be the woman society asks us to be, we risk becoming unrecognizable to ourselves.

It's time to rewrite the rules. To create a new 'normal' where women are celebrated not for their ability to endure things but for their refusal to. Where emotions aren't treated as liabilities but as the body's most powerful navigational tools. Where expressing your truth isn't an act of defiance, it's the baseline. Because when we stop explaining ourselves, when we stop apologizing for taking up space, we don't just reclaim our voices – we reclaim our health.

...

Now that you're conscious of the layers of shame that have shaped your adaptive self and suppressed your voice, the next step is understanding where all that unexpressed emotion goes when it doesn't have an outlet. In the next chapter, we dive into the biology of repression – how emotions that aren't metabolized don't just vanish but embed themselves into your body's fascia, nervous system, immune response, and hormonal rhythm. This is where the emotional body becomes the physical body. And it's where we begin to set you free.

Chapter 14
MACHINES REGULATE, HUMANS FEEL

'He had been wont to despise emotions: girls were weak, emotions... were weakness. But this morning he was thinking that being a great brain in a tower, nothing but brain, wouldn't be much fun.'

SHELDON VANAUKEN

In the late 19th century, Dr. Silas Weir Mitchell, a prominent American physician, devised the infamous 'rest cure'[1] – a treatment crafted explicitly for women diagnosed with 'nervous disorders,' which encompassed anxiety, depression, fatigue, and, perhaps most revealingly, any spark of creative or intellectual ambition.

The 'cure' consisted of confining women to their beds for weeks, even months, at a time, prohibiting them from engaging in any form of creative, intellectual, or emotional stimulation such as reading, writing, or socializing.

Charlotte Perkins Gilman, an accomplished writer and thinker, became one of Mitchell's patients when she began suffering from what we'd now recognize as postpartum depression. Instead of receiving the support her nervous system needed, she was subjected to Mitchell's oppressive regimen, which unsurprisingly, plunged her into even deeper despair.

However, rather than capitulate to the treatment's intended effect – emotional and creative docility – Gilman alchemized her suffering into a scathing critique of patriarchal medicine. Her semi-autobiographical short story 'The Yellow Wallpaper' (1892) chronicles a woman's descent into madness under the suffocating weight of enforced rest and emotional suppression.[2]

In 1960s Australia, a chemically induced iteration of the rest cure emerged: the painkiller Bex. Widely prescribed and marketed, primarily to housewives as a quick fix for the stress, exhaustion, and emotional strain of domestic life, its slogan was, 'A cup of tea, a Bex and a good lie down.' But beneath the soothing promise was a dangerous cost. Prolonged use of Bex led to cases of kidney disease, and countless women unknowingly sacrificed their health in a bid to silence their bodies' cries for rest, relief, and recognition.

What Are Emotions, Exactly?

While confining women to their bedrooms under the guise of treatment is no longer acceptable, today, women struggling with anxiety or depression are often prescribed medications which, while sometimes lifesaving, also serve as Band-Aids – numbing symptoms without addressing the root causes: structural inequality, emotional repression, and a chronic disconnection from their authentic desires, needs, and truth.

Instead of community or ritual, we now place women in sterile clinical rooms – or alone on Zoom calls – expecting them to heal in isolation. As the holistic psychologist Dr. Nicole LePera puts it, 'Indigenous cultures saw mental illness as imbalance – not a disorder.... They used community, ritual, and nature to heal. Maybe the primitive ones weren't them, but us.' Expressing our emotions (negative or positive) is met with shame, criticism, or dismissal, yet when our health suffers, the idea that stress, emotions, or trauma might contribute to conditions such as painful periods, PCOS, endometriosis, inflammation, or autoimmune diseases is often ridiculed or outright ignored.

This is a no-win situation in which acknowledging emotions leads to ridicule and suppressing them leads to suffering – both dismissed as personal failures rather than recognized as the consequences of a meticulously engineered system designed to control.

Make no mistake, our physical and mental disintegration is the intended outcome of a structure that fears the full force of empowered, expressive, and emotional women. But why do we fear women who are connected to their emotions? To arrive at the answer to that question, we must first understand what emotions offer us.

The Emotional Spectrum

When we talk about emotions, we're exploring them in their broadest, most expansive sense – as the ancient, intelligent forces that shape our lives, bodies, and relationships. We start with the familiar lineup: anger, fear, sadness, joy, contentment, and courage. These have been extensively studied and are known to be experienced and expressed across all human societies, regardless of language, geography, or cultural background.

American psychologist Paul Ekman labelled these as universal emotions,[3] noting through his groundbreaking research that they come with distinct facial expressions and physiological responses that can be recognized anywhere, from the streets of Tokyo to the plains of the Serengeti.

Then there are the more nuanced, layered states – shame, guilt, pride, gratitude – each shaped and shaded by the cultures we inhabit, the stories we tell ourselves, and the social structures we move through. It gets more complex when we consider the gnawing pull of hunger or the electric spark of sexual arousal. These are what psychologists refer to as 'drive states,' the primal urges that motivate behavior and push us toward survival.

But we can't forget the intangible experiences: The profound awe we feel under a star-strewn sky, the deep connection of spiritual inspiration.

It's only recently that science has begun to offer explanations for their biological foundations.

Not all emotions are treated equally by the brain, however. Emotions linked to stress – such as worry, fear, and anger – often receive priority in terms of attention and memory over feelings of happiness, peace, or even love. Why is this? Because from an evolutionary perspective, emotions are vital tools, helping us focus on what matters most. The nervous system is wired to remember emotionally charged experiences – especially those that signal danger or reward – so we can make better choices in the future.

Imagine an early human who knew which berry bush yielded sweet, nourishing fruit and which one left her doubled over in agony. The emotional impact of these experiences gave her a better chance of surviving (and passing on her genes) than someone who couldn't tell the difference as the memories were etched into her mind, guiding her behavior and, ultimately, the continuation of our species.

Neuropeptides: 'Molecules of Emotion'

This is where neuropeptides enter the story. Dubbed 'molecules of emotion' by pioneering neuroscientist Candace Pert in her groundbreaking book of the same name, neuropeptides are cell-to-cell signaling molecules that act as chemical messengers, transmitting emotional information throughout the brain and body.[4]

Now, it's tempting to think of emotions as a recent evolutionary development – a sophisticated side effect of our big, complex brains. But emerging research tells a different story – neuropeptide signaling actually predates the evolution of our Stone Age nervous system.[5] Yes, you read that right. Emotions are older than the nervous system.

This means that emotions have been guiding life on this planet for hundreds of millions of years. They're an ancient intelligence that not only secured our survival but powered our transformation. Emotions guide our decisions, fuel our creativity, and – most importantly – expose the fractures in systems that no longer serve us. They're the compass pointing us toward evolution both as individuals and as a species.

So, I ask you this: If emotions are this deeply rooted in the fabric of life itself – if they *predate* humanity – who are you to ignore them?

How Neuropeptides Work

Imagine your emotional state as water in a pool (your brain). When an emotion is triggered, a sudden surge of water spills over the edges of the pool. The neuropeptides released in response to that emotion flood into the bloodstream and flow through your entire system. From there, they travel into various tissues and organs.

Along the way, these neuropeptides bind to receptors in your heart, gut, endocrine (hormone) glands, and immune cells, influencing everything from your heart rate and digestion to hormone release and immune responses.[6] They alter the chemical environment of every cell they interact with, and this is why emotions are deeply felt throughout the entire body.

When it comes to processing and storing emotional experiences, we need to direct our focus to the hippocampus, the part of the brain responsible for learning and memory, as it's rich in receptors for messenger chemicals like neuropeptides and neurotransmitters. When an emotional event occurs, these chemical messengers surge through the brain, influencing the hippocampus and helping to encode the experience into long-term memory. In this way, these signals can act as emotional tags, marking specific experiences with unique biochemical signatures that make them easier to locate later.[7]

This explains why the faint scent of a familiar perfume, or the opening notes of a long-forgotten song, can instantly transport us back to a specific place in time. The neuropeptides released during the original experience help recreate the emotional and physiological state we were in, making the memory feel fresh, immediate, and alive.

Held in the Body

But here's where it gets even more fascinating. Neuropeptides don't just trigger emotional states; they *sustain* them. Unlike classic neurotransmitters (such as dopamine), which act quickly and locally, neuropeptides have a broader, longer-lasting impact.

Some neuropeptides can be changed in ways that help them last longer in the body. This means they can travel further and have effects in more places, not just where they were first released. This means that even if the cause of your emotion is gone, your body can stay in that emotional state for a prolonged period (hours, days, or weeks), as these circulating neuropeptides continue to influence various physiological processes.

This, of course, is wonderful in the context of positive emotions. When we experience joy, love, or excitement, the sustained release of neuropeptides allows us to bask in those feelings long after the initial event – strengthening social bonds and improving our physical health by reducing stress and promoting relaxation.

But this mechanism becomes damaging with toxic emotions such as unresolved anger, shame, chronic stress, or deep-seated grief. If we suppress or ignore these emotions, the neuropeptides associated with them continue to circulate.

In other words, emotions don't just fade away because we want them to – or because we ignore them. If we don't allow ourselves to acknowledge, feel, and express them, they become biologically embedded in our mind and body.

The Implications of Unexpressed Emotions

My father loves to remind me that I was a troublemaker as a toddler. Chuckling, he'll recount stories to friends of me stripping naked in the middle of the grocery store, fists pounding the floor, wailing at the injustice of not getting what I wanted – or, more importantly, what I needed.

I'm lucky. I come from a home filled with love and emotional connection, and my father is far more self-aware and nurturing than many men of his generation. And yet, these stories never sat well with me. They made me feel small and angry, and as I grew older, I realized that they were windows into a culture profoundly uncomfortable with women's emotions, from early life onward. They revealed how even the most loving homes are shaped by the cultural soil we grow in.

My dad went to an all-boys school, then an all-male college, and was trained in male-dominated institutions. Like many men, he was raised in systems that conditioned emotional suppression as strength, and was taught that girls who were loud, intense, or boundary-pushing were 'too much.'

But my frustration, my loudness, my refusal to be ignored were never a problem. They were a primal, intelligent response – a child asserting her boundaries, trying to get her needs met, demanding to be seen and heard. The real issue here is how quickly those emotions were dismissed by someone who loves me deeply, who values emotional connection, and who would call himself an advocate for my bold self-expression.

And it wasn't just limited to my frustration or anger. I'd squeal with happiness and shout with excitement, and those emotions, too, were met with 'Calm down,' or 'You're being too much.' Looking back, it's clear that my father wanted to protect me – acutely aware of how a girl like me, loud and unfiltered, would be treated in a world that doesn't know what to do with women who are fully expressed.

Wiring the Mind

By the time I reached adulthood, both ends of my emotional spectrum were blunted and I found myself sitting perennially in the middle – not too sad, not too happy, just muted enough to be manageable. And that's the tragedy that doesn't get enough of our attention. A lifetime of muting joy, excitement, and unbridled delight.

These weren't *my dad's* rules – they were the *system's* rules. And that's the point: You can be deeply loved and supported, and still absorb messages that teach you to shrink. Each of these early moments of dismissal or stifling are the building blocks of our neurological identity – they get etched into the architecture of our developing brains.

New tools have allowed us to study neuropeptides in greater detail than ever before, showing us their critical role in childhood brain development, influencing how neurons in the brain connect and how emotional information is processed.[8]

For me, it's painfully clear how this played out. As a child, being told to 'stop crying,' or being labelled 'hysterical' by my teacher was both emotionally scarring and neurologically formative. Each time this happened, neuropeptides flooded my system, reinforcing the idea that my emotions were too much – that I was too much.

Over time, this constant suppression altered my brain's neural pathways. The circuits that should have encouraged me to process and express my emotions were weakened, while those promoting emotional numbing and control grew stronger.

I didn't just *choose* to bottle things up, binge eat, and avoid conflict; my brain had been wired to do so through years of repeated experiences and neuropeptide signaling. Emotional expression had become a threat. But even in my silence, my body was paying attention. It was piling up every emotion I tried – consciously or not – to suppress. And it never forgot.

Our emotions, whether positive or negative, are energy in motion. They're designed to move through us, to be felt, processed, and to ultimately inspire us into action. But when we suppress our feelings, we create a kind of biochemical backlog.

How Suppressed Emotions Impact Our Health

In my case, the signs of emotional suppression were becoming impossible to ignore. Chronic tightness in my hips and lower back was my body's persistent whisper; a symptom I dismissed as the inevitable result of bad posture from sitting at a desk five days a week. But emerging research on the body's fascia – the connective tissue that surrounds every muscle, bone, and organ – revealed the deeper connection I'd been missing.

The skin was once heralded as the body's largest organ, but scientists now recognize that fascia holds that title. And fascia is far more than just the body's structural scaffolding. It's an intelligent, dynamic network of connective tissue with six times as many sensory nerves as its red muscle counterpart[9] that allows for almost instantaneous cellular communication throughout the body.

The Magic of Fascia

Fascia serves as a repository for emotional memory. A physical space where unprocessed emotions can be stored. It contracts and tightens in the presence of stress, grief, and fear, and over time, without body-based work of the kind that we're going to explore in Part III, chronic tension develops as the fascia tightens, thickens, and forms adhesions or knots that restrict movement and contribute to persistent pain.

And this physical imprint of emotional suppression doesn't just restrict movement – it reshapes the body's internal landscape, reinforcing cycles of pain, tension, and dysfunction. A growing body of research now shows that these unresolved emotional patterns don't just linger in the fascia – they contribute to broader physiological imbalances, manifesting in conditions like Major Depressive Disorder (MDD), anxiety, endometriosis, and menstrual irregularities – making it clear that what we hold in our bodies shapes our health in profound ways. Let's take a closer look at three of these conditions.

Major Depressive Disorder (MDD)

A fascinating German study assessed the fascia of 40 patients with MDD and 40 that had never been depressed.[10] They found that those with MDD had significantly stiffer and less flexible fascia in the neck and upper back regions, pointing to a tangible manifestation of their emotional distress.

A follow-up study on 69 MDD patients found that those who incorporated body-based techniques aimed at loosening the fascia (often with tools like foam rollers, massage balls, or even just the hands) experienced notable improvements in their mood and were also less likely to recall negative memories or dwell on negative thoughts compared to those who did not implement the treatment.

This may explain (in part) why exercise and other somatic practices have proven to be remarkably effective in treating depression. A comprehensive review published in *The British Medical Journal* in 2023 found that certain forms of exercise – especially dance – had stronger effects on reducing depressive symptoms than standard treatments such as selective serotonin reuptake inhibitors (SSRIs).[11]

But why dance? Unlike other forms of exercise, dance is inherently expressive. Through rhythmic movement, the body is given permission to express emotions that words often cannot: grief, anger, joy, and everything in between. It also stimulates the release of feel-good endorphins, which naturally elevate our mood.

Anxiety

Anxiety has deeply somatic (body-based) roots as well. A study in Spain looked at the effectiveness of myofascial release therapy (which works on the fascia around muscles) for a group of 36 adult patients with high levels of clinical anxiety.[12] Half of them received a 40-minute myofascial release session every week for a month, where four key areas were worked on for 10 minutes each: the abdomen, the chest (specifically the sternum), the base of the skull, and the earlobes.

The other half also attended sessions, but theirs didn't include the specific therapeutic techniques that define true myofascial release. The group that received true myofascial therapy experienced significant reductions in anxiety, decreased physical pain sensitivity, and fewer stress-related symptoms. Even more compelling was that these improvements lasted for six months post-treatment.

Endometriosis

This invisible illness affects 1 in 10 women worldwide yet it takes an average of seven to 10 years to diagnose. The emotional toll of living with constant, unexplained pain – while being dismissed, misdiagnosed, or outright gaslit – is immense.

A study published in the *European Journal of Pain*[13] examined 30 women with endometriosis-associated chronic pelvic pain and confirmed that their discomfort wasn't confined to the pelvic region. Instead they exhibited widespread myofascial dysfunction – tension and tightness in the connective tissues that extended throughout their entire bodies.

Their pain wasn't just localized to where the endometrial tissue grew; it was part of a full-body response in which muscles tensed, tissues stiffened, and the pain had become long-lasting and inescapable. A critical factor driving this cycle was pelvic floor muscle spasms – muscles so tight and contracted, they simply couldn't release.

This discovery begs a deeper, more important question: Why couldn't these muscles let go and relax? The answer lies beyond pure biology, in the realm of emotions.

The Effects of Stress

Chronic emotional stress leads to a phenomenon known as muscle guarding – a state where muscles remain in constant contraction, bracing against perceived threats. The body doesn't differentiate between the stress of a toxic relationship, the frustration of being dismissed by a doctor, or the trauma of living in a world that refuses to listen. It responds the same way: by tightening, holding, and preparing for battle.

Over time, this leads to myofascial adhesions (tight, sticky spots in the connective tissue), trigger points (painful muscle knots), and restricted blood flow. All these factors contribute to chronic pelvic pain, inflammation, and dysfunction – the key drivers of endometriosis.

But the ripple effect doesn't stop there. Myofascial dysfunction can exacerbate hormonal imbalances, ramping up cortisol production, contributing to estrogen excess, and disrupting immune function by fueling chronic inflammation.

These same mechanisms can also worsen conditions like PCOS, irregular periods, painful menstruation, PMS, and PMDD. Meaning that for many women, the root of their hormonal imbalances isn't just in their endocrine system – it's deeply embedded in how their bodies hold and process stress and unresolved emotions.

Ancient Wisdom, Modern Truth

While we're exploring the importance of healing from emotional suppression, it's worth turning to traditions that have long honored the body as a mirror of the soul. One of the most illuminating conversations I've had on this topic was with my dear friend and collaborator Mary Riposta, whose work sits at the intersection of modern neuroscience and Traditional Chinese Medicine (TCM) – two systems that, when brought together, paint a far more holistic picture of women's health than our current clinical frameworks allow.

Mary shared with me a core principle from TCM: When emotions, especially anger, are repressed, they don't just disappear, they stagnate. Specifically, they get 'stuck' in the liver, the organ responsible for maintaining the smooth flow of energy (*qi*) throughout the body. This condition, known as liver *qi* stagnation, is something Mary sees repeatedly in women who've internalized the need to be polite, perfect, and pleasing.

The liver also stores blood, which nourishes the reproductive organs, so, when its energy is stuck, symptoms often ripple outward into the menstrual cycle. From PMS and painful periods to PCOS, endometriosis, and fertility struggles, the body begins to carry what the voice cannot express.

In Mary's experience – and in mine – there's a consistent overlap between women dealing with reproductive health issues and those struggling to assert their boundaries, voice their needs, or give themselves permission to feel their rage.

In this way, TCM gives language to what many of us feel but can't explain: that our emotional lives and physical symptoms are not separate. Acupuncture, a key component of TCM, when paired with somatic work of the kind we'll explore in Part III, helps women finally make contact with the emotions we've had to suppress in order to survive – especially the ones we're never taught how to hold safely, like anger.

You Have to Feel It to Heal It

When the body becomes a battleground for unprocessed emotions, many of us unconsciously turn to the most immediate form of control we have: our relationship with food. We live in a culture obsessed with dieting, weight loss, and controlling our bodies, and every day we're bombarded with ads for pills, powders, and programs promising to 'fix' us. Solutions that would have rendered themselves obsolete long ago if they really worked. But they don't, because the problem is not our bodies.

When we fixate on thinness or controlling our appearance in other ways, we consume vast amounts of our precious and finite energy. This preoccupation keeps us focused outward, on the surface, instead of turning inward to confront the uncomfortable emotions lurking beneath. As long as we're pushing and striving to change our physical form, we remain conveniently distracted from the deeper work, the real work, of being present in our bodies and feeling the emotions we've been conditioned to fear.

But to undo this conditioning we must appreciate that it didn't start with us. The generations that came before ours weren't taught how to process their emotions. They watched their mothers swallow grief, suppress anger, and smile through suffering. They learned that being 'too much' came with consequences. So, they found ways to cope.

Marion Woodman, a Jungian analyst, captured this dynamic perfectly in her searing critique *Addiction to Perfection*. She described how individuals with restrictive eating disorders often long to be light, untethered from matter, to feel empty and clean – as if purging themselves of all emotional and physical weight. In the other camp, those who eat compulsively are trying to bury themselves, to anchor their existence in the physical world by adding layers of protection. Each extreme represents a different expression of the same fundamental struggle: a desperate attempt to numb emotions and escape the discomfort of inhabiting a body.

The body is the vessel through which we experience the world, the home for our feelings, and the container for our soul. Yet so many of us are spiritually and energetically disconnected from it. We live 'up high' in our mind, over-intellectualizing or dissociating from the sensations and emotions rooted in our flesh. We're taught to view our bodies as projects to be perfected rather than homes to be inhabited.

> ### *Pause for Self-Reflection*
>
> Use the journal prompts below to explore your thoughts, patterns, and experiences around food and emotions:
>
> - *In what ways have I used food to control or alter my appearance to avoid feeling something deeper?*
> - *Whose patterns around food did I unconsciously mirror (family members, friends, etc.) and what were they really trying to feel – or avoid feeling?*
> - *What emotions might be living underneath my relationship with my body and food?*

Food itself isn't the problem, then – it's the medium. It's the tool we've been handed in a society that refuses to let us feel. But if we could stop numbing ourselves – if we could sit in the discomfort of our emotions and listen to what our bodies are trying to tell us – we might discover a different kind of hunger. Not for food but for connection. For expression. For liberation. The women who came before us weren't given that choice. But we have been.

Emotional Sensitivity: Women's Superpower

What I hope is becoming very clear to you is that women's emotional sensitivity is one of our most formidable gifts. Neuroscience even confirms this. Women have stronger neural pathways connecting the amygdala (the seat of our emotional responses) to the prefrontal cortex (where decision-making and regulation occur), especially under social and emotional stress,[14] making us biologically wired to be perceptive, emotionally intelligent, and deeply attuned not only to our own internal landscapes but also to the emotional ecosystems around us.[15]

This is the intelligence that will shape the next iteration of our world, not artificial intelligence. AI can process data, optimize systems, and execute algorithms with precision, but it cannot feel. It can mimic emotion, but it will never embody it.

> *Women's empathy, intuition, and social awareness are sophisticated strategies that have allowed us to build communities, hold families together, and navigate relationships with grace.*

We're not machines. Machines regulate, humans feel. And in feeling deeply, we engage with the full spectrum of what it means to be alive. Our tears, our laughter, our heartbreak, and our joy are not glitches in the system – they are the threads that weave the rich, intricate tapestry of human existence. Healing, then, necessitates that we reclaim the fullness of our emotional spectrum. It's about coming home to ourselves – feeling, expressing, and honoring our emotions without shame or apology.

Our emotional complexity guides us through grief, points us toward joy, and connects us to the people, places, and experiences that give life its meaning. When we learn to trust in and stop apologizing for the depth of our feelings, we will reclaim our humanity.

The world needs women who are willing to feel deeply, to empathize profoundly, and to lead with emotional intelligence. The world doesn't need less of us. It needs more. More empathy. More intuition. More courage to build a life that doesn't just *look* good on the outside but feels rich, authentic, and deeply satisfying on the inside.

...

In the concluding chapter of Part II, we begin the shift from awareness to embodied action. You'll discover that you're not just an indicator of a broken system but the initiator of a new one. Healing isn't where the story ends – it's where leadership begins.

Chapter 15
WOMEN – FROM INDICATORS TO INITIATORS

'The most dangerous thing a woman can do is learn how to love herself. And that's when they start to fear her – because she's finally free.'

UNKNOWN

In Chapter 4, we explored the idea that women are an indicator species – that our bodies are often the first to signal when the environment has become unlivable. From menstrual disorders to chronic fatigue, autoimmune disease to infertility, our bodies are sending signals that the system in which we live is out of balance.

But that's only one part of the story. Because when a woman starts to heal and reclaim her power, something else happens. She doesn't just stop at signaling what's wrong. She starts showing what's possible. She becomes a model of a new way forward.

As she listens to her body and speaks her truth, she evolves from indicator to *initiator*. From the one sounding the alarm, to the one building the new blueprint. From the one carrying the symptoms, to the one restoring the system.

A Force of Nurture

During the COVID-19 lockdowns, my search for healing led me through books on trauma, somatic therapy, and cellular memory. But one day, out of the blue, I found myself drawn to a podcast about forests. Not my usual genre, but something within told me to *listen*.

The episode featured Dr. Suzanne Simard, Professor of Forest Ecology at the University of British Columbia in Canada and the author of *Finding the Mother Tree: Discovering the Wisdom of the Forest*. Raised in a multi-generational Canadian logging family, she'd grown up watching trees being felled en masse, their remains carted away as nothing more than timber for profit.

Forests, she was told, were economic assets. Something to manage. To control. To extract from. But as she pursued her research, Dr. Simard began to see the forest differently. She discovered that trees are not isolated competitors fighting for survival but interdependent beings constantly communicating – sharing resources, warning of threats, and supporting one another through intricate underground fungal networks (confirming beliefs that Indigenous communities have long held).

At the center of these networks are the Mother Trees – ancient, deeply rooted elders that nourish the young, guide the forest, and stabilize the ecosystem. They give carbon to saplings that can't yet survive on their own. They send biochemical signals to warn others of drought, disease, and danger. They are wisdom-keepers. Lifelines. Guardians. 'Trees don't compete. They communicate,' Simard says. 'They send distress signals about drought and disease, and other trees alter their behavior when they receive these messages.'[1]

That image stuck with me, and I realized that women – especially powerful, embodied women – are the Mother Trees of humanity. When we're unwell, it's not just a personal issue, it also reflects something deeper in the culture. But when we're well, we're not just thriving, we're supporting life around us.

We become a stabilizing force. A source of safety. A leader of change. This is what it means to be rooted in power.

> *When we stop seeing ourselves as isolated individuals and recognize our collective role as nurturers, connectors, and culture-shapers, we'll shift more than our own lives.*

When a woman is rooted in her truth and aligned with her biology, she no longer adapts to systems that harm her. She starts creating systems that support her, and others, simply by modelling a new way of existing.

When you live differently, people feel it. We all have something called mirror neurons – specialized brain cells that help us understand and respond to the actions, emotions, and states of others. They allow us to 'mirror' what we see, often unconsciously – forming part of how children learn, how empathy works, and how cultural norms are transmitted.

So, when a woman chooses to rest when she's tired, to set a boundary without apologizing, or to speak her truth instead of performing, it impacts those around her on a biological level. Her presence gives others permission to show up differently, too. This is how women become change-makers – not through pressure or perfection, but through presence. Through modelling a different kind of power.

Building the New System

As we've explored in this book, the old system is falling apart. Anything built on domination, disconnection, and extraction was never designed to support life. It was built for control, not for care. And now, it's reaching its breaking point. We're seeing it in our overburdened health systems, our toxic work culture, our lonely relationships, and our degrading environment. Burnout, imbalance, and dis-ease are everywhere because the system itself is unsustainable.

But something else is emerging. And powerful women are helping to lead it. Its foundation is matriarchal – not meaning that women dominate but that the values of care, connection, and collaboration are put back at the center. It's a system that recognizes the intelligence of cycles. That prioritizes nourishment over depletion. That sees rest as a requirement, not a reward.

This new system also makes space for the sacred masculine to rise in its healthy form. We still need structure, direction, and protection – but not the kind that dominates or suppresses. The masculine in this system serves life instead of trying to manage it. It protects what's sacred rather than silencing what's sensitive. It partners with the feminine rather than trying to overpower it. As Mary Wollstonecraft wrote in *A Vindication of the Rights of Woman*: 'I do not wish women to have power over men; but over themselves.'

> *Pause for Self-Reflection*
>
> *If you were to fully step into the identity of an initiator – a woman who heals herself and becomes living proof of what's possible – what shift would you want your presence to create in the world?*

That's the kind of power this new system is built on – not domination, but self-ownership. This is not softness as weakness – this is softness as strategy. A woman who is rooted in herself doesn't need to control others. She leads by example.

She creates change simply by choosing not to abandon herself in a world that taught her to. And we do this work knowing that not every woman is free to do so... yet. In many cultures, communities, and households, stepping into full expression is still dangerous. Power is still punished. Visibility is still met with violence.

And so, we must become so rooted in the truth of who we are and what we are capable of that our very presence reshapes the cultural soil. We must be so undeniable in our wholeness that the world reorganizes itself around our existence. This is the work our bodies have been demanding.

...

You've remembered who you are. Now, it's time to rise into who you came here to be. Part III will guide you through reclaiming the power you hold from the systems that have suppressed it. This is where your personal healing becomes a blueprint for collective change.

Part III
RISING FROM THE ROOT

This is where everything you've remembered becomes real.

Not in theory, but in your body.

Not someday. *Now.*

You've questioned the systems.

You've faced the stories.

You've reclaimed parts of yourself that were never broken, only buried.

Now, it's time to rise from a place of deep inner safety.

Through clearing stressors, nervous system work, subconscious reprogramming, and my ThetaSomatics™ method, you'll rebalance the four foundational hormones – cortisol, insulin, dopamine, and oxytocin – and restore safety to your mind and body.

This is where awareness becomes action.

Where knowing becomes living.

Where the woman reading this stops waiting and starts leading.

Where you begin to live from a new baseline. One where stress doesn't spiral you, your body feels like home again, and your biology supports your brilliance.

This is the moment you start rising – from the root.

Chapter 16

ROOT RESTORATION: CREATING MIND AND BODY SAFETY

'Your body is the piece of the universe you've been given, and it's where it all begins.'

GENEEN ROTH

At this stage in the journey, you've peeled back the layers and traced the roots of disconnection through systems that were never built with your well-being in mind. You've learned to decode your symptoms as signals. To see your behavioral and relational patterns not as failures but as protective adaptations. And to finally recognize your body not as a problem to fix but as a source of profound intelligence.

So, how do we bring it all together? How do we go beyond insight and awareness and create lasting transformation – the kind that's rooted in physiological and psychological safety?

The Five Core Roots of Safety

In the following chapters, we'll be working with the second stage of the Root Restoration Framework you were introduced to in Chapter 8.

This process is the bridge between everything you've uncovered so far in the book and everything you're now ready to embody. It integrates the science, the somatics, and the soul of this work into clear, actionable steps for transformation.

Through nourishing what I call the five core roots of safety – authenticity, conscious safety, environmental safety, historical safety, and unconscious safety – you'll begin to reduce your allostatic load (stress bucket) and rewire the invisible conditions that shape your nervous system, your hormones, your thoughts, your behaviors, and ultimately, your experience of life.

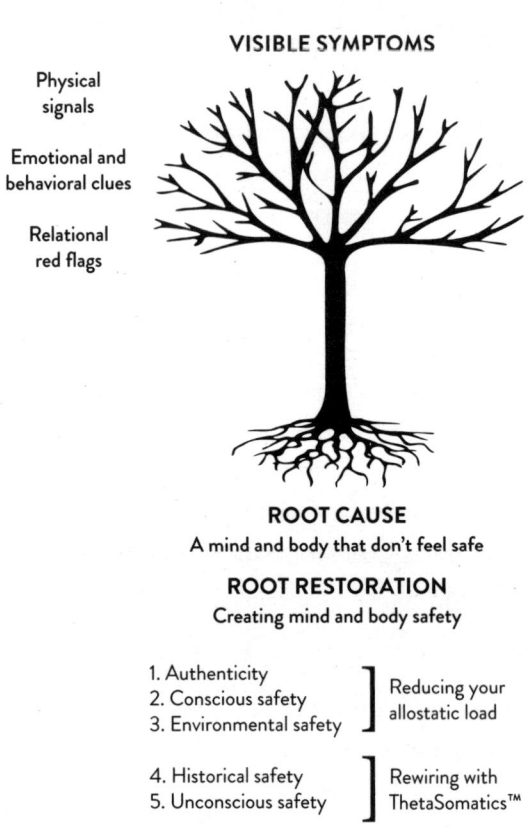

The Root Restoration Framework

Together, the five core roots help to restore a sense of safety to the mind and body. Here's an overview of what they encompass:

Root 1: From Inauthenticity to Authenticity

Coming home to who you are beneath the roles, rules, and reward systems. Reclaiming your wholeness, even when it's messy, emotional, powerful, or wild.

Root 2: From Conscious Stress to Conscious Safety

Clearing mental, emotional, and physical space and expanding your capacity to hold more without burnout.

Root 3: From Environmental Stress to Environmental Safety

Restructuring your inner and outer environments so they support your biology, not sabotage it. From your home to your habits, your cycle to your schedule – everything gets to align.

Root 4: From Historical Stress to Historical Safety

Beginning the ThetaSomatics™ process of releasing inherited trauma, stored emotions, and the unconscious imprints passed through generations.

Root 5: From Unconscious Stress to Unconscious Safety

Rewiring the beliefs stored in your subconscious mind. This final root helps you move from the survival loop to self-trust, so that your actions are no longer dictated by fear or lack but by worthiness, clarity, and possibility.

How to Approach Root Restoration

When we first recognize the need for deeper emotional release, nervous system regulation, or confronting our subconscious beliefs, it's natural to feel eager to dive in. This work is life-changing and once you see the patterns clearly, the desire to shift them can feel urgent. But your nervous system doesn't respond to pressure, it responds to safety.

Your nervous system expands and contracts. This natural rhythm, known as pendulation, means that as you begin to clear old patterns, your mind may challenge you and your body may cling to familiar comforts. That doesn't mean you're doing it wrong – it means your system is recalibrating. Moving through this stage becomes far easier when you're well-resourced with rest and nourishment.

Please be aware that you don't need to implement everything in this part of the book at once. Some of what you'll find may be brand new to you. Other elements may feel familiar – perhaps you're already practicing some of them, consciously or not. Wherever you're starting from is perfect. The goal isn't to overwhelm yourself with tasks, but to familiarize yourself with the practices and techniques first, then come up with a plan that works for you.

Part of reclaiming your power means giving yourself permission to go at your own pace. So, as you read the following chapters, I encourage you to treat them as a blueprint rather than a checklist. That said, here's a suggestion for how you might approach Root Restoration.

Weeks 1–5: Reducing Your Allostatic Load

Chapters 17–19 To integrate this work in a way that's sustainable, the first step isn't to do more, it's to do what's most supportive. And that means reducing your allostatic load – the cumulative stress on your body's systems.

This phase is about creating capacity in your nervous system and lifting pressure from your mind and body. You'll focus on reconnecting with your authenticity, clearing stressors, and creating inner and outer environments that support healing.

Weeks 6–8: Rewiring with ThetaSomatics

Chapters 20–21 Once your system feels safer, you'll be ready to explore the deeper subconscious and somatic rewiring work offered here. These chapters walk you through core ThetaSomatics™ techniques and other somatic practices to release stored trauma and reprogram adaptive beliefs at the root.

Week 9 Onward: Your New Lifestyle

At this point you'll understand how all the pieces fit together. This is where the Root Restoration work becomes a way of life, and you can begin tailoring it to your unique rhythms and routines.

Trust Your Timeline

Transformation takes time and repetition. Research suggests that it can take around 40 days of consistent practice for the brain to begin favoring a new habit or belief – not just cognitively but emotionally. That's when the nervous system starts to register this new way of being as safe. And when safety clicks into place, identity can begin to shift. So, if at any stage you feel tempted to quit, ask yourself: *If I knew this would work out* (because it will if you keep going), *what step would I take right now?*

Concerned that you don't have enough time? One of the greatest lies ever sold to women is that there's never enough – time, energy, space, or love. The truth is that time is not the issue – fear is. Ask yourself: *What am I avoiding by convincing myself that I don't have enough time? What would happen if I slowed down, prioritized myself, and embraced simply being?*

Healing doesn't require dramatic overhauls – it thrives in the micro-moments of intentional choice. You don't need more time – you need permission to stop rushing, to let go, to celebrate the small wins, and to put yourself first.

Not sure when to start? Start *now.* You don't require a diagnosis to begin this work. You don't need someone else's validation to know that something's off. Waiting for external permission only keeps you in limbo, doubting your inner wisdom. You're the expert on your body. Trust yourself.

In the next chapter, we begin the first root: authenticity. This is where you remember who you were before you were taught who to be.

Chapter 17
ROOT 1: AUTHENTICITY

'Sometimes just being yourself is the radical act.'
ELAINE WELTEROTH

A forest isn't beautiful because all the trees are the same. It's beautiful because they aren't. Each grows according to its own blueprint – some stretching tall toward the sun, others waving their branches low across the earth. Some bloom or bear fruit early; others take their time. We don't question which one is 'right' or 'perfect.' We don't look at one tree and tell it to be more like the one next to it. But we do this to ourselves.

The field of interpersonal neurobiology shows us that healing doesn't happen in isolation. It happens in relationship. As you'll recall from Chapter 11, authenticity is one of your two core needs. Your nervous system longs for you to feel fully seen, known, accepted, and loved exactly as you are. And just as a tree depends on the richness of the soil it grows in, you'll only truly thrive when the cultural soil surrounding you is fertile – when the environments, relationships, and communities you root yourself in nourish your full expression.

Authenticity is a biological necessity. Your nervous system will feel safe and regulated when you feel secure in being seen for who you truly are. The more freedom you have to be yourself, the more resilient and radiant you become. But if you invent a persona in order to be liked, you'll never feel truly loved. If you constantly manage perceptions, you'll always feel isolated. Ultimately, your nervous system doesn't really care *what* you're doing, just *why* you're doing it.

Feeling Safe to Be You

So, when you deny your authenticity or spend all your time in places that don't celebrate it, your body registers it. The moment you realize that you'll never be the perfect fit for everyone and release the need to be universally liked, is the moment you set yourself free.

Below are the three most important questions you'll ever ask yourself. I encourage you to take a moment to journal your answers with courage and curiosity. Be honest with yourself.

1. Am I truly choosing my life? Am I living in alignment with my deepest truth, or am I simply meeting the expectations of others?

2. How much of what I believe, value, and do is actually my own?

3. How much has been shaped by the need to please, belong, or be 'enough'?

For many women, the truths that emerge can feel both unsettling and even frightening – because they reveal a life that isn't entirely their own. Remember, your health, relationships, success, and overall well-being depend on your ability to live authentically and feel safe in your truth.

The goal isn't to make everyone like you – it's to magnetize the people who genuinely resonate with your story and self-expression. But you must share your light so that others can find it. There's a community out there activated and inspired by your true essence. People who will thrive in your presence precisely because of who you authentically are, not who you pretend to be. The clearer and bolder your authenticity, the faster those who aren't aligned with you will naturally fall away, creating space for your true community to find you.

And the *right people* won't just merely like you; they'll trust themselves more deeply around you. By being yourself, you grant permission for others to reclaim their own truths and step out of the system. So, the question you need to be asking yourself isn't: *What if people don't like me?* It's: *What if the people who are meant for me never find me because I'm too busy trying to be liked by the ones who weren't?*

Getting to the Core of Who You Are

I know just how easy it is to mistake who you've been told to be for who you really are. For years, I believed my 'authentic' self was ruthlessly ambitious and hyper-independent. The woman in the red power suit with a slicked-back ponytail, thriving in high-pressure environments. I sourced my joy from perfection, external validation, late nights drinking with friends, and being recognized for my success.

When I finally slowed down enough to explore my subconscious, I reconnected with the version of me that had been buried beneath years of pressure and trauma. The girl who spent hours lost in her imagination. The girl who created for the sake of creation, who danced, performed music with her friends, was spontaneous, and never once questioned whether she was 'enough.' That was me before I learned who I was *supposed* to be.

The following practice, the Authenticity Audit, was inspired by the intention behind Dr. John Demartini's Value Determination Process. It's designed to help you to strip back layers of conditioning and reconnect with your true values, desires, and self-expression.

After reflecting on your responses to 15 key questions, you'll choose four personal truths, or 'authenticity anchors,' that will serve as a decision-making filter for every opportunity, relationship, and habit. You'll no longer need to look to someone else to tell you what's right for you. Instead, your inner clarity will become your guide through turbulence, darkness, doubt, contraction, and expansion. You don't have to hustle for worthiness or prove your value anymore. You simply are. And from that place, every decision, every relationship, and every next step becomes clear.

The Authenticity Audit

Now, it's time for you to get to the core of who you truly are by completing your Authenticity Audit. For the best results, do this exercise first thing in the morning (before checking your phone), when your brain is still transitioning through the slower theta and alpha brainwave states. This dreamy, in-between phase gives you easier access to your subconscious mind, before the noise of the day kicks in.

In this state, the barrier between your conscious and subconscious mind is thinner, making it easier to access clarity and truth. Other ways to shift into this deeper state of awareness include listening to binaural beats music (which plays two slightly different frequencies in each ear), completing a meditation, or doing a breathwork practice.

I also recommend completing the audit by hand in a journal; writing is a great way to access your subconscious because it slows down your thinking just enough to bypass the mental noise and drop into deeper, more intuitive layers of awareness. This way, you're not just answering questions – you're allowing buried insights, forgotten memories, and core desires to rise to the surface.

Step 1: Answer 15 Key Questions

Find a pen, a sheet of paper or your journal, and head to a quiet spot where you won't be disturbed for 20–30 minutes. Read through the questions below and then write down your 'top four' answers to each one:

1. **Perfect day:** When imagining your perfect day, what activities and experiences would you include that bring you the most joy?

2. **Desires:** If there were no financial constraints and you were going to treat yourself, what experiences/indulgences/treats would you choose?

3. **The future:** When daydreaming about your future, what specific subjects, objects, people, or experiences do you visualize?

4. **Childhood essence:** Looking back to your childhood, what were the activities, games, books, or places that brought you the most joy and curiosity?

5. **Internal dialogue:** What do you find yourself thinking about the most?

6. **Impact:** Where do you think you've made the most positive impact on others?

7. **Passions:** What topics or subjects do you find yourself talking about most often when socializing – for example, at dinner parties or lunch with friends?

8. **Joy:** Reflect on the last 12 months. When did you experience pure joy, awe, or bliss? What were you doing, and who were you with?

9. **Big vision:** Reflecting on your big vision for your life, what do you hope to achieve?

10. **Life force energy:** What activities, hobbies, or passions make you feel the most alive?

11. **Sources of inspiration:** What do you find yourself researching or saving the most? For example, books, podcasts, magazines, Pinterest, Instagram, TikTok, or screenshots.

12. **Time:** What activities take up most of your time and energy when you're just being yourself?

13. **Authentic abundance:** What do you spend most of your money on?

14. **Organization:** Looking at your calendar, environment, work, finances, fitness, family, and social life, where in your life are you most organized?

15. **Reliability:** In which areas of your life are you the most reliable, disciplined, and focused? For whom and what, and when, do you consistently show up?

Please keep in mind that neural processing in the brain happens at remarkable speeds, so trust whatever comes up for you instinctively and don't overthink it. This is about your authenticity. Don't write down what you think you 'should' but instead be radically honest with yourself.

Step 2: Identify Your Authenticity Anchors

Now look over your answers. You'll likely notice repetition – perhaps even a lot of it. You might have written variations on the same idea, such as 'spending time with people I love' or 'going out for brunch with my friends.' If you step back, you'll start to see the patterns.

Your task now is to distill these insights into four core words – your 'authenticity anchors' – and write a short explanation under each one. These anchors will keep you grounded in the truth of who you are so that you stop outsourcing your authority when you feel lost or unsure.

Examples of authenticity anchors from my clients include peace, depth, play, growth, belonging, freedom, family memories, expression, adventure, trust, stillness, curiosity, ritual, faith, movement, imagination, service, leadership, and flow. And below are the authenticity anchors I landed on after my first Authenticity Audit:

Wonder: Learning, new experiences, and feeling inspired. For example, reading books, exploring new scientific research, developing my spirituality, visiting museums and galleries, listening to music, watching a sunset, or reading poetry.

Community: Expressing myself honestly in relationships, whether it's at the local coffee shop where the staff know my order, with aligned friendships, or my family. Creating and participating in activities that make me feel connected to others, whether online or in person.

Creativity: Self-expression in all forms, including content creation, writing books or poetry, fashion, singing, painting, or brainstorming ideas. It could even be as simple as cooking dinner or creating a new Pinterest board.

Self-care: Exercise I look forward to, such as yoga and Pilates; healthy food, my beauty rituals, taking time for myself; and, crucially, slowing down when my body is calling for rest.

My anchors have evolved since I wrote these, and that's to be expected. Authenticity is a living, breathing thing. As we shed old identities or move through new seasons of life, our core words will shift too. As I do with my clients, I encourage you to revisit this audit annually, perhaps on your birthday, at the start of a new year, or whenever you feel out of alignment.

Daily Practice: Authenticity in Action

Keep your four authenticity anchors where you can't ignore them – on your fridge, on the first page of your journal, your phone lock screen, or bathroom mirror. Whenever you're choosing how to spend your time, money, or energy, check in with them, asking: *Is this aligned with who I truly am? Or am I defaulting to old patterns?*

Expressing your authenticity doesn't have to be a grand gesture. While I've now built my entire life around my anchors – even leaving London to live in Spain so I can walk on the beach every day – when I was still working in consulting, I read poetry on my lunch break, scrolled through Pinterest on the Tube journey home, and bought an adult coloring book to do in the evenings. Even the smallest acts of alignment boost dopamine and oxytocin, enhancing feelings of joy, safety, and momentum.

Of course, your authentic self-expression may challenge people. Be ready for a little bit of pushback. The world is conditioned to resist those who refuse to conform. When you're misunderstood, criticized, or pressured to shrink, your instinct may be to adapt, withdraw, or over-explain. This is where boundaries become essential. And that's exactly where we're headed in the next chapter.

But first, remember this: being firm in your authenticity doesn't have to be loud or aggressive. Let it be the quiet, steady, rooted presence of someone who knows who they are. No justification. No dilution. No apology.

When you own your truth, you become magnetic. The people, opportunities, and experiences meant for you will begin to find you. And if you experience intense resistance, remember that it's the ones who push back the hardest who feel your power the most. By identifying and using your four authenticity anchors, you create a decision-making filter for your decisions and lifestyle that keeps you grounded in who you are, even when the world tries to pull you off course.

* * *

Now that you're clear on who you are and what's important to you, you can begin the process of eliminating stressors to expand your capacity for the deeper work that lies ahead.

Chapter 18
ROOT 2: CONSCIOUS SAFETY

'An unexamined life is not worth living.'
SOCRATES

Conscious safety is the kind of safety you know you're seeking – such as feeling respected in a relationship or having control over your schedule. Cultivating conscious safety therefore begins by eliminating stressors that are within your control: the boundaries you need to set, the energy leaks you can plug, and the obligations that are fully within your power to release. It's time to shift into deeper integrity with your time, choices, and focus.

The Life Audit

In the following exercise you'll reflect on where in your life things feel aligned, where they don't, and where small, intentional shifts could create profound relief. Sometimes, it's not that we're doing *too much* but that we're doing too much of what's no longer in resonance.

You don't need to make dramatic changes overnight (though if you feel called to, please do go for it). Instead, try to focus on cultivating *clarity*. This is a chance to pause, zoom out, and identify where your current energy and life force are leaking.

Step 1: Evaluate 12 Areas of your Life

Grab your Authenticity Audit, a pen, a piece of paper or your journal, and find a quiet space where you won't be interrupted for 20 to 30 minutes. Review the 12 key areas of your life below by responding to the questions that follow them:

1. Business/career
2. Finances
3. Mental health
4. Media and social media consumption
5. Physical health
6. Friendships
7. Romantic relationship
8. Family
9. Hobbies and creativity
10. Learning and personal growth
11. Adventure and travel
12. Home and environment

Question 1: On a scale of 1–10, how satisfied are you with this area of your life?

Question 2: Why did you give the area that score? Make your answer more specific by responding to the following three questions:

- What's going well in this area of your life?
- What isn't going well in this area of your life?
- How can you add more elements of authenticity to this area (use your Authenticity Audit here).

Here's an example:

Physical health – score 6/10

- **Going well:** I'm working out consistently 3–5 times a week for 45 minutes. I get out for a 3-mile walk regularly after work and I usually hit the stand goal on my Apple watch.

- **Not going well:** I wish I had more friends to work out with, and I wish I could make it more fun. Most of the time I dread going to the gym and drag myself along on my walks.

- **Authenticity Audit add-on:** Take a workout class (such as Zumba) and ask my friends to join me for yoga on the weekend. I'm going to find some new podcasts to listen to on my walks so that I look forward to them.

Step 2: Detox, Delegate, and Ditch

Your energy is a precious currency. You wouldn't hand out your money carelessly, so why do you give away your energy so freely? It's time to honor where you spend it and consciously decide what stays (detox), what shifts (delegate), and what goes (ditch).

Look over your Life Audit. Where are you overcommitted? What tasks, relationships, or obligations feel like a constant drain? Make your way through each of the 12 areas of your life, creating a list of action steps that fit into three groups:

Detox

In this group, put anything that *has* to stay in your life but could be streamlined – made lighter, easier, or more enjoyable. Here are some examples:

- Instead of the constant stream of text messages in my girls' group chat as we try to coordinate plans to meet up, I'll set up a standing monthly 'girls' night' (say, the first Thursday of every month).

- Instead of cooking dinner from scratch every night, I'll create a weekly menu with the kids and batch cook on Sundays. That way, I'll have nourishing food in the freezer without the daily stress of preparing it.

Delegate

Here, list what can be shared, outsourced, or handed off. Examples might be:

- Trust my junior colleague to compile the monthly client reports so that all I need to do is review and send them.

- Hire a cleaner once a month to deep clean the house instead of spending every Saturday doing it all myself.

Ditch

For this group, think about what you're holding on to out of guilt, habit, or obligation:

- Gracefully decline invitations to events I don't feel aligned with, instead of forcing myself to go, out of FOMO or politeness.

- Unfollow influencers on social media who make me feel like I'm not doing enough, and curate my feed with people who inspire and uplift me.

- Replace doomscrolling with bloomscrolling.

Daily Practice: Conscious Safety in Action

Some shifts – like declining events you don't want to attend, unsubscribing from emails that clutter your inbox, or automating bill payments – can be implemented immediately (and I encourage you to do so now, to build momentum and enjoy a hit of dopamine). Others, such as setting boundaries in relationships, restructuring your workload, or navigating long-standing commitments, require more time, energy, and capacity.

That's okay. The Life Audit is a living tool that will evolve with you. As you grow, so will your boundaries. What feels impossible to action today will eventually become a non-negotiable to which you don't give a second thought. Your daily practice is simply to commit to noticing where your energy is leaking and making small shifts when you can.

Here are three golden rules to living in a way that protects your energy:

1. **Your energy is your responsibility.** No one else is responsible for managing your burnout or depletion. The more you protect your energy, the more you'll have to give where it truly matters and build an authentic, aligned life for yourself.

2. **If it's not a full-body yes, it's a no.** Your body knows before your mind does. Pay attention to what expands you and what contracts you. To what gives you energy and what leaves you depleted.

3. **No is a complete sentence.** You don't need to justify, soften, or over-explain. Express yourself, don't explain yourself. The people who have their own boundaries and respect you will honor your boundaries.

Of course, saying no, prioritizing yourself, and setting clearer boundaries may stir up discomfort. Guilt, hesitation, or the fear of disappointing others may surface – especially if those around you have benefited from your over-giving. This is normal.

But every time you pause to check in with yourself, every time you say no when you once would have said yes, every time you protect your energy without justification, you expand the capacity of your nervous system to hold this new level of self-love.

And once you begin implementing the deeper ThetaSomatics™ work in Chapters 20 and 21, you'll stop fighting yourself into holding boundaries. You'll *become* the kind of woman whose body recognizes boundary-setting as safe, loving, and necessary. The more you practice, the more easeful it becomes – not because your circumstances change, but because *you do*.

...

Now that you've cleared space and begun aligning your external life with your internal truth, it's time to go even deeper. In the next chapter, we shift the focus from what you do to what surrounds you – your physical environment, your daily habits, your food, your light, and your exposure to toxins.

Because no matter how much inner work you do, if the environment you live in is working against your biology, your body will stay overwhelmed. We'll also look at reconnecting with what brings you pleasure and embracing your cyclical nature.

Chapter 19
ROOT 3: ENVIRONMENTAL SAFETY

*'Take care of your body,
it's the only place you have to live.'*

Jim Rohn

One cold January morning during lockdown in London, as I stepped out of a steaming shower, I caught a glimpse of myself in the fogged-up mirror. Immediately, the familiar script of self-criticism began replaying in my mind: 'I'm fat. Ugly. Not good enough.' Despite diligently attending Pilates classes and strictly adhering to a wholefood diet, I still felt bloated, drained, and disconnected from myself.

I'd recently been prescribed antidepressants after a brief consultation with a physician I'd waited six weeks to see. A vague diagnosis based solely on my low mood, without any real enquiry into my lived experience. The pills sat unopened on my desk.

I'd spent an enormous amount of time, money, and energy chasing every new diet, wellness trend, or healing protocol, hoping each would finally deliver the breakthrough I longed for. But that morning, it finally dawned on me that no amount of discipline, willpower, or physician appointments could overcome the deeper truth of what was really happening in my body.

I didn't need more rules – I needed to strip things back to basics and tune out the overwhelming noise.

Our minds and bodies evolved over thousands of years to thrive under certain fundamental conditions, and I'd been massively overcomplicating things. I realized that true transformation wouldn't come from micromanaging my symptoms or overthinking every solution; instead, it would come through creating environments – both internally and externally – that truly aligned with my biology.

Getting Back to Basics

This chapter will guide you back to your body's foundational settings, the essential pillars of healing that your system already recognizes. Regulating blood sugar, reducing toxin exposure, reconnecting with nature, reclaiming your natural cyclical rhythms, and prioritizing pleasure will significantly reduce strain on your mind–body system.

This will free your energy and resources for healing and self-repair, giving you the clarity, space, and confidence to engage deeply in the transformative work in Chapters 20 and 21.

Reset Your Internal Clock

Every day, the natural cycle of sunrise and sunset cues critical functions in our bodies. For example, at sunrise, natural light signals your brain to kickstart the release of cortisol to boost your alertness and wake you up. Then as daylight wanes and the sun sets, your body responds by reducing cortisol production and producing melatonin, the sleep hormone that prepares you for a restful night.

However, our constant exposure to blue light from screens (laptops, phones, TVs) in the evening is confusing this natural rhythm, tricking the brain into thinking it's still daytime. This makes it harder for you to fall asleep and prevents your body from getting the deep, restorative sleep that it needs for healing, hormone regulation, and cognitive function.

And this is just *one way* in which changes to light exposure subtly disrupt your body's ability to function optimally. So, here are two small adjustments to your daily routine that can have a profound impact on your internal clock:

1. **Get morning sunlight exposure:** Aim to get outside in natural light within the first hour of waking, even if it's just for 5–10 minutes. If you live in a place where mornings are dark, consider investing in a sunrise-simulating alarm clock.

2. **Reduce blue light exposure after sunset:** Minimize your screen time in the evening, choose candles over bright lights, or wear glasses that block blue light at least two hours before bed – my favorite come from Bon Charge.

Seriously, these small tweaks are powerful – give them a try.

Regulate Your Blood Sugar

Our metabolism was designed to work in harmony with the natural world. Our ancestors thrived on whole, single-ingredient foods – rich in fiber, balanced in carbohydrates, abundant in healthy fats, and with protein and minimal sugars – providing steady energy and supporting the body's natural hormonal rhythms. Today, our food landscape looks drastically different, filled with ultra-processed, sugar-laden, and nutrient-depleted foods that disrupt our metabolic balance.

A key player in this delicate system is insulin, which acts as the body's metabolic regulator. In essence, insulin's primary job is to shuttle glucose (sugar) from the bloodstream into cells, where it can be used for energy or stored for later. When this system functions optimally, energy levels remain stable, cravings stay in check, and your hormone hierarchy (*see page 47*) thrives.

However, constant blood sugar spikes – caused by frequent consumption of refined carbohydrates, sugary foods, cycles of restriction, bingeing, and stress (thanks to cortisol's impact on insulin) – lead to insulin resistance, a state where cells become less responsive to insulin's signals. This not only disrupts energy and mood but also contributes to weight gain, inflammation, and hormonal imbalances – for example, elevated estrogen and PCOS.

Below are three simple yet powerful strategies to support your insulin levels.

1. Eat Foods in the Optimal Order

At mealtimes, by consuming fiber (vegetables) first, and carbohydrates and sugars last (after protein and fats), you can reduce your overall blood sugar spike by up to 73 percent and insulin spike by 48 percent.[1] In 2018 research from Stanford University in the US also demonstrated that eating a sugary breakfast can send glucose levels soaring to levels as high as in people with diabetes, even in those who don't have the condition.[2]

Our bodies are especially sensitive to glucose and sugar- and starch-heavy foods in the mornings (e.g. sweetened iced coffees, acai bowls, or fruit smoothies). Savory choices such as eggs with vegetables, the classic English breakfast with protein and fats, or omelets offer much better blood sugar control.

2. Prioritize Protein

Include sources of plant or animal protein – such as eggs, chicken, or legumes – at every meal to support muscle health and hormone production (protein provides the building blocks for hormones). Your protein needs will differ based on your age, body size, activity level, and lifestyle, but a general recommendation for women is 0.75–1oz (20–30g) of protein with each meal, three times a day, aiming for a total of 2–3.5oz (60–100g) of protein daily.

3. Build Muscle

Muscle is one of the most powerful tools for regulating blood sugar. Think of your muscles as glucose storage tanks – the more muscle mass you have, the more efficiently your body can clear excess glucose from your bloodstream by using it for energy.

This improves insulin sensitivity, stabilizes blood sugar levels, and reduces the risk of insulin resistance. Incorporating strength training into your routine 2–3 times per week can have a profound impact on your metabolic health. If you're new to resistance training, bodyweight exercises or resistance bands are a great place to start.

Reduce Your 'Toxic Load'

While not all of us will be able to eliminate our exposure to chemicals, we can take plenty of active steps to minimize it and support our body's natural detoxification processes. Protecting your health and hormone balance starts with simple shifts – here are five to try:

1. Filter Your Water

Investing in a high-quality water filter is one of the simplest yet most effective ways to reduce your exposure to harmful chemicals like PFAS (so-called forever chemicals that resist breaking down), chlorine, pesticide residues, and heavy metals.

Pharmaceutical hormones – particularly synthetic estrogens from birth-control pills and HRT – have also been detected in water supplies worldwide. While municipal water treatment plants remove many contaminants, they don't always filter out endocrine-disrupting compounds (EDCs), which can interfere with natural hormone function. Research has even shown that fish stocks in British rivers are in serious danger of collapse because male fish are changing sex in response to female hormones released into the water.[3]

2. Ditch Plastic

Store food in glass or stainless-steel containers instead of plastic to reduce your exposure to Bisphenol A (BPA), an industrial chemical used in plastic manufacturing. Avoid reheating your food in plastic or drinking out of plastic water bottles – heat accelerates the release of these toxins.

3. Choose Natural Products

When it comes to what you put on your body and bring into your home, nature knows best. For cleaning, simple ingredients like apple cider vinegar, lemon juice, baking soda, and castile soap are surprisingly powerful. They cut through grease, lift stains, and disinfect without exposing you to harsh chemicals.

For beauty and personal care, start replacing products with natural alternatives as you finish them – especially for things you use daily such as shampoo, conditioner, makeup, perfume, and deodorant. This also applies to clothing and furniture. Many synthetic fabrics shed microplastics that end up in the dust we breathe. Where possible, choose natural fibers like cotton, linen, silk, and wool.

4. Eat Natural Food

Choose single-ingredient, organic produce to cut pesticide exposure by up to 90 percent in just a week. If that's out of budget for you, clean supermarket fruits and veggies effectively instead: fill a bowl with water and add 1 teaspoon of baking soda for every two cups of water. Soak your produce for 10–15 minutes, then give it a good rinse (baking soda helps remove pesticide residues and dirt better than water alone). For tougher skins (such as on apples), gently scrub with a brush while soaking.

Choose hormone- and antibiotic-free meats such as pasture-raised or wild-caught fish to avoid hidden disruptors. If these are beyond your budget, look for lean cuts, trim excess fat (where toxins often accumulate), and incorporate more plant-based proteins such as lentils or beans.

5. Reconnect with Nature

Your body and nervous system are designed to thrive in blue and green spaces where the air is fresh, the light is natural, and the rhythms are slow.

Step outside daily, even if it's just for a few moments. Feel the sun on your skin. Listen to the birds. Walk barefoot on the earth. Breathe deeply.

If you live in a city, carve out time to visit parks or green spaces, and when planning holidays or getaways, consider centering them around nature, water, and open landscapes that naturally regulate your nervous system. You don't need to uproot your life to reconnect – just create small, intentional moments where you let the natural world hold you.

Daily Practice: Back to Basics in Action

You may be doing a lot of the things above already, or perhaps this chapter has caused you to reconsider your whole lifestyle. No matter where you're at, it's important to remember that small shifts make a big difference, especially when done consistently. Think of this as a gentle recalibration, not a perfection project.

Begin by writing a list of the new habits you're going to implement and choosing just one to focus on this week. That's it. Maybe it's stepping outside for five minutes of morning light. Maybe it's adding a little more protein to your breakfast; buying some blue light-blocking glasses; or finally switching your plastic containers for glass. Then next week, add another habit.

I've focused on a mix of the most common and overlooked environmental stressors that impact women globally. However, if you suspect that you may be grappling with deeper drivers such as nutritional deficiencies, histamine intolerance, mold exposure, mitochondrial dysfunction, gut health imbalances, chronic inflammation, heavy-metal toxicity, or metabolic challenges, I encourage you to explore these further with a trusted practitioner.

And always consult a physician to rule out more serious concerns, such as tumors, autoimmune disorders, structural issues, or genetic conditions that may be disrupting your body's natural rhythms.

Prioritizing Pleasure

Women are biologically designed for pleasure (hello, oxytocin!) – it's central to our well-being, and our anatomy confirms it. Consider the clitoris: an organ equipped with around 8,000 nerve endings devoted solely to the female orgasm. By comparison, the penis, which serves reproductive, urinary, and pleasurable functions, contains roughly half that number, about 4,000 nerve endings.

Unsurprisingly, while the clitoris appeared in medical texts as early as the 16th century, it was largely omitted from mainstream anatomical literature and discussions. It wasn't until Australian urologist Dr. Helen O'Connell's groundbreaking research in 1998 – and her comprehensive imaging studies in 2005 – that the clitoris was fully mapped and recognized as a significant internal structure.

Given how recently even medical professionals became fully aware of the clitoris's anatomy, it's understandable that many women have felt disconnected from their own pleasure. Women's sexual enjoyment is still frequently portrayed as indulgent, shameful, or even dangerous. This suppression isn't accidental; it directly aligns with patriarchal structures designed to disconnect us from our instincts, silence our desires, and undermine our trust in ourselves.

You won't experience pleasure if you don't feel safe, which is why so many women struggle to orgasm or cultivate a healthy libido. And when you're disconnected from your pleasure (and consequently, your womb–throat power pipeline (*see page 141*), you feel depleted and dysregulated, and you're more easily controlled.

Of course, pleasure extends beyond sexuality – it's deeply connected to sensuality, a richer and broader experience. As my friend Henika Patel expresses so beautifully in her book *Sensual: Connect Deeply, Express Freely, Love Deeply*, sensuality involves fully engaging with life through all our senses, nurturing a profound connection to our bodies, surroundings, and emotions beyond just sexual contexts.

Pleasure is both medicine and essential information. It's one of the most direct paths to healing, hormonal balance, and emotional resilience. By embracing pleasure through sensual self-touch, mindful and intentional movement, dedicating time to activities and people you love, or simply savoring everyday experiences (the warmth of your coffee, the sun on your skin, the softness of your sheets), you signal safety to your nervous system through the release of oxytocin.

This explains why a lack of orgasms can cause significant stress in the body. The hormonal cascade that follows orgasm reduces inflammation, balances cortisol levels, improves sleep, and recalibrates your nervous system to its restorative, parasympathetic state.

Daily Practice: Embrace Pleasure

Reclaiming your power isn't only about healing past wounds – it's equally about expanding your capacity for joy. You were never meant to merely survive your life – you were meant to *deeply feel and experience it*. The more you allow yourself to embrace pleasure, the more capacity you develop to hold beauty, love, intimacy, and joy without shrinking or shutting down.

Create Your Pleasure List

Pleasure doesn't have to be grand or time-consuming – in fact, the more accessible it is, the better. Write a list of 10 small, nourishing things to do that will help you feel grounded, soft, alive, or connected to your body as you move through your day. Here are some ideas:

- Slowly sipping your morning tea or coffee
- Self-touch (whether a sensual caress or a grounding massage with coconut oil)
- A bath with music, candles, or essential oils
- Cuddling your pet
- Fresh sheets and a slow stretch in bed

- Dancing in your underwear to your favorite song
- Wearing beautiful clothes or jewelry just for yourself
- Taking a long walk with an inspiring podcast
- Listening to music
- Making love

Check out ways to boost your oxytocin levels (*see page 104*) if you need more inspiration – but most importantly, tune in to what *actually* feels good to you.

Express Your Pleasure

For most of my life, when I was engaging in something pleasurable (such as drinking a delicious matcha latte) I'd rush through it, muting or minimizing my expression. So, I encourage you to consider this: Do you allow yourself to moan with delight when you taste something exquisite? Do you let pleasure ripple through you when you dance, when you stretch, when you make love? Or do you cut it short, rush toward the end goal, suppressing sensation before it has a chance to expand?

The more you allow pleasure to flow through you, the more oxytocin you produce. And when you start allowing yourself to linger in the feeling, to *savor* it, you send a powerful message to your body: *I'm safe enough to receive these positive emotional experiences.* This is how you cultivate the conditions for healing and self-repair, while also rewiring for joy and creating a stronger baseline of safety.

Aligning with Your Biological Blueprint

Whether you're in your reproductive years, are navigating perimenopause, or have moved beyond menstruation altogether, this section will help you root your daily life in the truth of who you are biologically, reconnecting you with the adaptability, resilience, and intelligence embedded within your cyclical rhythms.

By working *with* your body rather than against it, you can begin living in a way that finally *feels* good and sustainable. Because when you stop forcing yourself into a linear, masculine model of productivity and start living cyclically, you begin to access a deeper current of energy and intuition that's always been there.

Cyclical Living: the Reproductive Years

Learning to live in sync with your menstrual cycle is a practice that takes time, observation, and self-compassion, so start small. Begin by noticing how you feel each week: your energy, mood, cravings, libido, and emotional needs. Track your cycle and symptoms using a journal or one of the many great apps available (that don't sell your data without consent); I personally love Moody Month and Clue.

If you're on hormonal birth control and are thinking about transitioning off, you can begin cultivating cyclical awareness now by syncing with the moon. Use the new moon to represent menstruation and the full moon to represent ovulation. This gentle rhythm helps you reconnect with your body's natural ebb and flow, even before your own cycle returns. For trans women, following the moon's phases in this way can also be a deeply affirming practice – a way to honor your body, embrace feminine energy, and root yourself in cyclical wisdom.

Of course, aligning with your biology may require you to make different choices in how you work, how you move, how you relate, and how you rest. You might even realize just how unsupportive your current lifestyle is. But the change doesn't have to be dramatic.

Start by reclaiming your power in small but significant ways: Plan creative projects or social events during ovulation, build in rest and reflection during your luteal (premenstrual) phase, honor the natural ebb and flow of your libido. In Chapter 18, we cleared space mentally, emotionally, and physically to prepare for this lifestyle shift. So now, you have the capacity to create new habits that help life feel more like flow than friction.

Work with the Phases of Your Menstrual Cycle

As we explored in Parts I and II, your hormones, energy, and nervous system shift rhythmically across each phase of your cycle. So, by tailoring how you eat, move, fast, and connect to match these changes, you work with your body rather than against it.

Fasting, in particular, sends strong signals to the body. In the wrong phase, it can mimic famine – triggering a stress response and disrupting hormone production. But when done in alignment with your hormonal landscape, it can be supportive.

Menstruation (Winter)

Approximately days 1–5

- **Exercise:** Prioritize rest and gentle movements such stretching, foam rolling, or yoga. You're more prone to injury now, so allow your body the time it needs to recover.

- **Nutrition:** Warm, comforting foods are incredibly supportive now. Choose iron-rich foods (grass-fed beef, spinach), root vegetables, and fresh ginger tea to soothe any cramps.

- **Fasting:** This is the optimal time for longer fasts if desired, as both estrogen and progesterone are at their lowest. You can try intermittent fasting (14–16 hours) or an even longer fast if it feels right for you, as your body is naturally in a state of reset.

- **Superpowers:** Your intuition is heightened. Reflect on the past month and set intentions for the next cycle. It's a perfect time for journaling and internal work.

- **Sex:** Some women prefer rest, while others enjoy the intimacy of period sex. If it feels right for you, lean into the deeper, loving connection it can bring. Honor whatever your body needs, without judgment.

Follicular (Spring)

Approximately days 6–14

- **Exercise:** This is your best time for new challenges. High-intensity workouts like strength training, HIIT, or running feel great as your energy builds. Try that new class you've been curious about!

- **Nutrition:** Focus on healthy fats and omega-3 fatty acids (avocado, salmon, nuts) to support growing follicles. Add in fiber-rich foods such as raw carrots and cruciferous vegetables (broccoli, kale) to aid the proper breakdown of estrogen.

- **Fasting:** Intermittent fasting works well here (12–15 hours), but keep fasts shorter and opt for earlier dinners rather than skipping breakfast. Your body handles fasting well during this phase as it's preparing for ovulation.

- **Superpowers:** Creativity and problem-solving are at a peak. Use this time to start new projects, brainstorm ideas, and tackle complex tasks.

- **Sex:** Your libido will start to increase but it might still be gentle and exploratory – not everyone wants wild, kinky sex straight after their period (if you do, go for it!). Otherwise, enjoy intimate, affectionate sex with lots of foreplay, mirroring the building hormonal surge.

Ovulation (Summer)

Approximately days 15–17

- **Exercise:** You're at peak energy here so go for your toughest workouts: heavy lifting, sprints, or power yoga. Push yourself, but listen to your body if it signals to slow down.

- **Nutrition:** Anti-inflammatory foods are key. Include leafy greens, berries, and fermented foods such as kimchi. Support your liver with detox teas (milk thistle, dandelion).

- **Fasting:** Keep fasting shorter (12–14 hours), especially if you're trying to conceive, have lower progesterone levels or high stress levels. Focus more on hormone-supportive eating rather than longer fasting.

- **Superpowers:** Your communication, charisma, and confidence are off the charts. This is the perfect time for important meetings, networking, first dates, having difficult conversations, and asking for a promotion.

- **Sex:** You're in your most fertile window, and if your hormones are balanced, it'll show! This is the time to make the most of your high libido and have more adventurous and playful sex (if that calls to you).

Luteal/Premenstrual (Autumn)

Approximately days 18–28

- **Exercise:** In the early luteal phase, you can stick to resistance training. But tune in to your body and as your energy dips, switch to more restorative activities such as Pilates, stretching, foam rolling, or gentle walks.

- **Nutrition:** Your body needs more calories now, so focus on nutrient-dense, fiber-rich foods. Load up on magnesium-rich choices (such as dark chocolate and leafy greens) to help with PMS symptoms. Fresh ginger tea can ease cramps, reduce inflammation, and support digestion. You're also much more sensitive to blood sugar fluctuations, so rely on the aforementioned hacks when leaning into your cravings.

- **Fasting:** Avoid long fasts now because your body requires extra nourishment for hormone production. Instead, try shorter fasts (10–12 hours), focusing on balanced meals with plenty of protein, healthy fats, and complex carbs to keep blood sugar stable.

- **Superpowers:** Your analytical skills shine here. Instead of using them to pick apart your life, turn your attention toward refining projects, planning, and tying up loose ends. Embrace the urge to organize and prepare for the next cycle.

- **Sex:** Sensual and slow is the name of the game, and remember, it's normal to have less cervical fluid and be less 'wet,' so rely on non-toxic lubricants to support you. Cravings for intimacy might shift to a deeper, emotional connection. This is the time for love-making that feels nurturing and grounding.

Over time, this way of living will become second nature to you. You'll feel your energy stabilize and your creativity flourish, your hormones rebalance, and your self-trust deepen. You'll know, intuitively, what you need and when – and when it comes to pleasure, you'll feel far more confident expressing your desires because you'll *know* what turns you on in each phase of your cycle.

Cyclical Living: Menopause and Beyond

Cyclical living doesn't end when menstruation does. It evolves. During perimenopause, or the menopause transition, your hormonal landscape begins to shift dramatically as estrogen and progesterone levels become more erratic, which can trigger changes in sleep, mood, energy, and metabolism. This is not a 'decline.' It's a biological recalibration – an initiation into a new rhythm that requires care, curiosity, and compassion. Try the following during perimenopause and menopause:

- Embrace the rhythms of this transition by tracking your symptoms rather than your cycle. What patterns do you notice around energy, mood, sleep, digestion, and libido? Let that data inform your self-care.

- Support your nervous system by building in more recovery time – whether that's resting between workouts, pausing throughout your day, or creating space for emotional processing. Reduce conscious stressors (the Life Audit on page 191 will be very supportive) and focus on eating more magnesium- and protein-rich foods.

- Prioritize gentle, grounding movement over high-intensity workouts if you're feeling depleted. Honor what your body needs.

Postmenopause, your hormonal landscape levels out into a new baseline. Many women find that their intuition sharpens, their need for external validation fades, and their desire for authenticity becomes non-negotiable. Consider these intentions as anchors for this next powerful season of your life:

- You may no longer bleed, but your body is still deeply responsive to rhythm and ritual. Trust your own energy – this stage of life invites deeper self-trust and more intentional living.

- Focus on nourishment, both physical and emotional. Build routines that support quality sleep, creative expression, sensuality, and strength.

- Surround yourself with people and practices that ground and expand you.

In many ways, postmenopause is a rebirth. With hormonal shifts no longer prioritizing fertility, a new kind of life force becomes available – one rooted in truth, vision, and legacy. You become the oracle. The truth-teller. The woman who no longer apologizes for taking up space, who asks for what she needs, and walks away from anything that drains her. It's a time when many women step into leadership, become spiritual mentors, birth new creations (businesses, art, activism), and claim their fullest self-expression.

• • •

Now that you've created more capacity by lightening a significant allostatic load (stress bucket), it's time to explore the weight of what's been passed down: The emotional imprints, beliefs, and unresolved trauma that live in your nervous system and cells. It's time to reclaim historical safety and begin your ThetaSomatics™ journey.

Chapter 20
ROOT 4: HISTORICAL SAFETY

*'Most of us have become separated from our natural,
instinctual selves – in particular, the part of us that
can proudly, not disparagingly, be called animal.'*

PETER LEVINE

In my first two years at university in Sydney, Australia, the city's nightlife was my sanctuary. The bassline in my chest, bodies moving in sync, sweat and laughter blurring into one dizzying, neurochemical-fueled wave. I was always one of the last ones standing, chasing the next hit of aliveness – not always from substances, but always from sensation.

In hindsight, I see it clearly: I was chasing oxytocin, dopamine, and endorphins – the natural highs I was starved of. The dance floor was giving me what real life couldn't. I felt free. Unshackled. Weightless. But then the morning came. And my body, ever honest, told a different story. Tears would catch me off guard – silent, sudden, slipping down my temples in the stillness of a Pilates cooldown.

One morning, as I lay on the mat, eyes closed, my instructor saw what I hadn't yet named. She simply said, 'You know, what you're doing out there – it's not just escape and numbing. It's release.' A proud queer woman, she then paraphrased writer and activist Dan Savage's reflection on the peak of the AIDS crisis: We would bury our friends in the morning, protest in the afternoon, and dance all night – the dancing is what kept us in the fight.

We're built to move, shake, tremble, and purge. Our bodies are the archives of our individual, collective, and intergenerational lived experiences, where unresolved emotions imprint themselves on neural circuits and cellular structures alike. This chapter is all about reclaiming the wild, instinctual, primal intelligence of your body – the part that knows how to complete the stress response cycle (*see page 90*), process, release, and heal, if only given the chance.

Cultivating Historical Safety

Creating historical safety means teaching your body that it's safe *now*. That *your lineage* is safe now. That you no longer need to brace or wait for the next impact. This is where we begin to apply the healing method I've developed, ThetaSomatics™, which blends evidence-based somatic practices (like rocking, shaking, and yoga-informed movement) with original modalities that I've created through years of personal and professional exploration (you'll experience one of these later).

We start with simple movement practices because, for you to fully benefit from the subconscious rewiring work coming in the next chapter, we must first teach the nervous system and fascia how to let go of the past and move through the discomfort of showing up differently in the world. Releasing historical stress and cultivating historical safety happens in two distinct phases. Before we get started, let's look at what these involve.

Phase 1: Release the Old. First, we must shift the backlog of emotional debris and stress that's weighing you down. In this phase, you'll use simple, yet very effective, somatic techniques to clear out unprocessed emotions and stored tension, allowing you to naturally shift into regulating your nervous system.

Phase 2: Regulate to Rewire. As you release the weight of the past, your internal space and capacity begin to expand. This makes it much easier to recognize when you've encountered a stressor, slipped into nervous system dysregulation, and begun moving around the survival loop (*see page 125*). Rather than spiraling, you'll be able to catch it in real time – and pause.

This newfound awareness allows you to begin interrupting the survival loop before it gains momentum, rewiring your response over time. And from that space, you'll be ready to go deeper: to meet the subconscious belief driving the response and begin the healing work that follows in the next chapter. And best of all, you'll find yourself shifting into nervous system regulation practices intuitively when the following happens...

- Your baseline state shifts. You move through your days with a deeper sense of calm and ease.

- You're no longer ruled by old emotional patterns. When you're triggered, there's now space to pause, to choose, and respond differently.

- You can track the regulation of your nervous system. You notice when you're slipping into dysregulation and course-correct before it fully takes hold.

- Instead of feeling stuck in your emotions, you experience them as temporary, fluid, and manageable.

- Instead of just surviving, you start planning your future from a foundation of self-trust, confidence, and stability.

So, get ready to finally *let go* of the past and embrace pleasure and joy because you have the skills to handle whatever challenges your internal sense of safety.

Phase 1: Release the Old

Somatic work influences the body's stress response through various neurophysiological pathways. When practiced consistently, these targeted movements support the recalibration of systems affected by chronic stress, helping to restore hormonal balance, reduce cortisol, and alleviate stress-related disruptions to the menstrual cycle.

Note that when you're working on releasing the old, you may feel an immediate shift, or the release might come hours or days later – through vivid dreams, new memories surfacing, spontaneous tears and bowel movements, unexpected emotions (such as joy, euphoria, grief, rage), or a deep sense of relief and freedom.

If nothing surfaces at first, that's also completely normal. If your body has been in a state of suppression or dysregulation for years (or generations), it may take time to trust that it's truly safe enough to let go. This isn't something to force or fix. Your body knows exactly what to do and it will release at the right time. Your only job is to be consistent.

Pick Your Somatic Practice

Below is a menu of somatic practices you can use in Phase 1; if you're new to this type of work, I recommend that you pick just one practice to explore at a time so you can notice which ones feel the most supportive to your body. If you have the capacity for deeper releasing work, you might choose 2 or 3 of the practices to explore over the course of a week.

> *Pause for Self-Reflection*
>
> Before you pick which practice you want to experiment with, check in with yourself. Answer the following questions in your journal:
>
> - *What sensations are present in my body? (Tightness, heaviness, tingling, numbness?)*
> - *What emotions are present? (Anger, frustration, contentment, excitement?)*
> - *Where do I feel tension or resistance? (Neck, shoulders, chest, heart space, fists?)*

Note that after a release, your nervous system needs time to recalibrate – without this step, you risk bypassing the full impact of the work. Support your system by prioritizing grounding activities like walks in nature or deep rest, revisiting the self-reflection prompts above to note any shifts, and hydrating and nourishing your body to help clear stress-related chemicals.

A note on timings: Perform your chosen practice(s) for the recommended 'release durations.' If you're short on time or simply not in a place where you want to process heavy emotions, you can still begin establishing a conversation with your nervous system by using the 'safety durations' instead. These tell your body: *Hey, I'm here now. You don't have to brace anymore. It's safe to soften into safety.*

Dance

Dance is one of the most instinctual and powerful ways to release historical stress. This type of spontaneous movement activates the limbic brain (responsible for processing emotions) and encourages the completion of the stress response cycle. As Katherine Dunham, a pioneering dancer, anthropologist, and ethnographer who studied the role of dance in different cultures around the world reminded us, we dance because we must. Dance is an essential part of life.

Here's how to begin connecting with dance as a practice of release and remembrance:

1. Select a song that feels right. Maybe you need something cathartic, slow, or emotional, or maybe you need something light, silly, or playful.

2. Stand in a space where you feel safe and uninhibited and move freely, using your whole body. Close your eyes if it's safe to do so and let your body lead.

3. Bring special attention to your hips – for example, try circling them slowly, swaying side to side, or incorporating deep, rhythmic undulations.

Release duration: 9–15 minutes (3–5 songs)

Safety duration: 2–3 minutes (1 song)

Rocking

This is among the earliest forms of nervous system regulation we encounter as we're gently swayed in the womb by our mother's inhales and exhales. Rocking is a rhythmic motion that stimulates the parasympathetic nervous system, fostering a profound sense of safety and relaxation. Research shows its power in diverse contexts, from improving heart rate variability and emotional regulation in children with severe motor and intellectual disabilities,[1] to easing mood and alcohol cravings in military veterans using rocking chairs.[2]

Cycle through the following three rocking techniques. You can enhance the experience by playing calming music (such as binaural beats) to deepen relaxation. This is a wonderful grounding practice for the morning or a soothing wind-down before bed.

You'll know your body has shifted into the parasympathetic state when you naturally yawn, sigh, exhale deeply, feel a stomach-gurgle, or even experience spontaneous tears – all signs that your nervous system is settling into safety.

- **Windscreen wipers:** Lie on your back with your arms beside you, feet flat on the floor about hip-width apart and knees pointing to the ceiling. Gently rock your knees from side to side like windscreen wipers. Move at a pace and range of motion that feels comfortable to you – these don't have to be big movements.

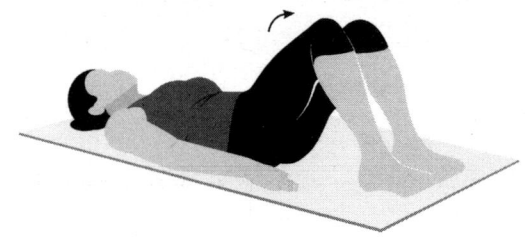

- **Ankle windscreen wipers:** Lie on your back with your legs straight, feet relaxed and toes pointing to the ceiling. Gently rotate your ankles from left to right, playing with the speed and range of motion. Allow the movement to engage your legs and hips.

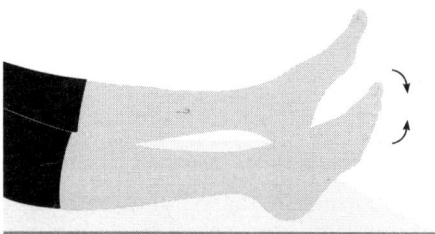

- **Side-lying rocking**: Lie on your left side in a loose fetal position, with your knees bent comfortably in front of you. Rest your head on your left arm and place your right hand gently on the floor in front of your chest for support. Begin to softly press into your hand, allowing your upper body to rock forward and back in a slow, rhythmic motion like a cradle. When that feels complete, switch to your right side and repeat.

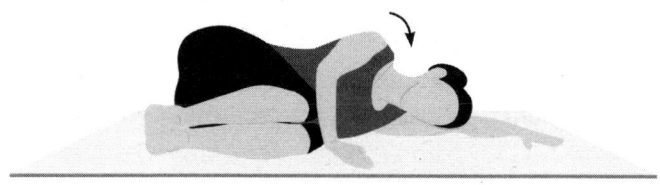

Release duration: Spend 5 minutes on each movement (2.5 minutes per side for the side-lying rocking)

Safety duration: Spend 3–5 minutes on any single rocking technique

Gypsie, one of my clients in Australia, shared with me how rocking helped her PCOS: 'I've reached eight months of consistent ovulation and semi-regular periods with my PCOS (between 25 and 30 days)! My skin remains clear, with the odd pimple when my period approaches. My period symptoms have also begun to slowly reduce. It's crazy how simple rocking can create such a regulated mind, and you begin to find time in the day to bring yourself back to a state of calm and crave a sense of peace. It's wild to think of the dysregulated and lost woman I was at the beginning of the year.'

Somatic Shaking

Animals shake instinctively during or after experiencing stress to discharge excess adrenaline and cortisol, and reset their nervous systems. We were designed to do the same. I suspect that one of the reasons Taylor Swift can hold her overwhelming amount of fame and attention is because, as her song says, she can literally 'shake it off'!

You'll know you've had a release when you yawn, sigh, cry, feel emotions rising, or experience a sense of lightness. Here's how to do somatic shaking:

1. Stand with your feet shoulder-width apart.
2. Begin by shaking your hands and wrists, then your arms, shoulders, hips, and legs in turn.
3. Eventually, your body will begin shaking on its own. This might take time and practice, so stay patient.
4. Let the shaking intensify if it feels good, then gradually slow down.
5. Use your breath to exhale out tightness and tension.

Release duration: 5–10 minutes

Safety duration: 1–2 minutes

Hip Opening and Sound Activation

The hips and pelvis are among the deepest reservoirs of emotional memory in the body, particularly for grief, shame, and anger. When we experience fear, stress, trauma, or emotional repression, the psoas muscle (often called the muscle of the soul), which connects your lower spine to your thigh bone, contracts, holding tension long after the triggering event has passed.

To effectively release hip and pelvic tension, you must engage both movement and sound. Vibration activates the vagus nerve, signaling safety to the nervous system and opening the womb–throat axis, or power pipeline (*see page 141*), enabling profound emotional release.

Move through these hip-opening positions, using cushions or yoga blocks to support you if you need modifications as these can be intense stretches. Integrate sound by humming deeply or sighing audibly and slowly. Lower, guttural tones resonate best in the pelvic area.

- **Pigeon pose:** This provides deep release for the outer hips and psoas. From all fours or downward dog, bring your right knee toward your right wrist and extend your left leg behind you. Keep your hips as square as possible, using a cushion under your right hip if needed. Fold forward from the waist, rest your arms or head comfortably, and breathe in deeply, letting out a sound on your exhales. When you're ready, change sides.

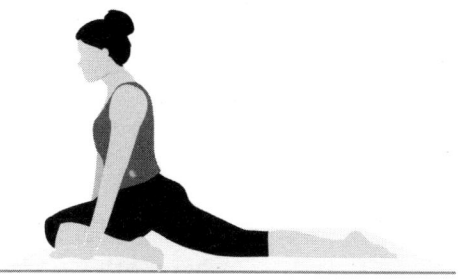

- **Seated butterfly:** This pose helps release tension in the pelvis and inner thighs. Sit with the soles of your feet together and your knees bent out to the sides. Hold your ankles or feet and gently bounce your knees up and down, like the wings of a butterfly. This rhythmic movement encourages your pelvis to soften and invites gentle release through the hips and groin. Breathe in slowly and let out a sound on your exhales.

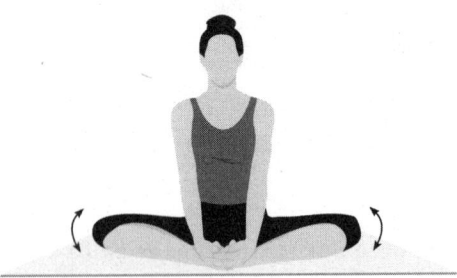

- **Low lunge:** This deeply targets the hip flexors and pelvic fascia, helping to open the front of the body and release stored tension. Step one foot forward into a lunge position, lowering your back knee to the ground. Keep your front knee stacked over your ankle and gently sink your hips forward. Your arms can be above your head, down by your sides, on your front thigh, or even resting on blocks – whatever is comfortable. Breathe into the stretch, letting out a sound on your exhales. Change sides when you're ready to move on.

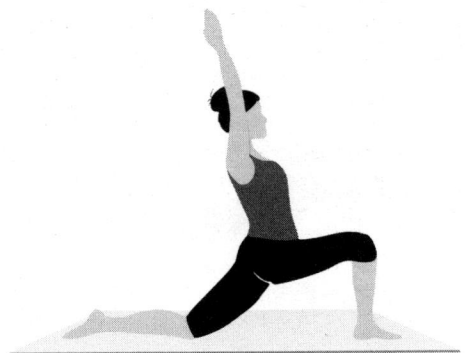

Release duration: 3–5 minutes per position (e.g. 2.5 minutes per side for a total of 5 minutes)

Safety duration: Choose one position and stay there for 1–2 minutes

Progressive Muscle Relaxation (PMR)

PMR is a simple technique that involves systematically tensing (or tightening) and then relaxing (or releasing) different muscle groups in the body. It signals to your nervous system that it's safe to let go, and it enables you to release tension, enhance body awareness, return to the present moment, and calm your mind.

PMR is especially effective for those who hold tension in their jaw, shoulders, or stomach without realizing it and can be done even in the middle of a stressful event (I used to tense and release my toes and feet during long work meetings).

- Find a quiet space (perhaps your bed, during a break at work, or even your car).
- While seated or lying down, methodically tense and then relax one muscle group at a time. Start at your face and work your way down to your feet. Inhale slowly through your nose and tense the muscles in one area for 5–10 seconds. Then exhale slowly and fully through your mouth as you release the tension completely. Let your breath carry the sensation of *letting go*.

Release duration: 10–15 minutes

Safety duration: 2–5 minutes

Releasing Anger

In my last year at boarding school, we were given time slots to march into the middle of the sport's field and scream as loud as we wanted to release the stress, anger, and anguish of final exams. It was effectively a structured, school-approved rage release. Genius.

And yet, almost none of the girls did it. We were much too embarrassed to be seen expressing that much emotion. I really wish I'd given it a go because it turns out that controlled anger-release not only feels really good but is also incredibly effective. Here are a few ways you can do it safely and privately:

- **Scream into a pillow** (if full vocal release feels too big, start by humming loudly and work up from there).
- **Scream underwater** – for example, in the ocean, a bath, or a pool. This is shockingly effective, but don't forget to come up for air!
- **Punch a cushion/pillow/mattress** over and over again.
- **Grab a cushion/pillow** and slam it down on your bed repeatedly.
- **Stomp your feet** if you feel a surge of energy in your legs. This can be anger, frustration, or simply a need to discharge built-up tension through movement.

Release duration: 3–5 minutes

Safety duration: 1–2 minutes

Deep-release duration: 7–10 minutes. This extended session for significant stored anger allows the anger to move in waves – you may start intensely, slow down, then feel another wave rising. Try cycling through the different methods above. You'll find that your body starts generating heat – maybe you'll feel sweaty, flushed, or even shaky. This is a good sign. It means energy is moving.

Afterward, bring yourself back to a state of calm with slow, deliberate breaths, a cool shower, or lying down with your hands on your belly. Notice how your body feels. Lighter? Softer? More spacious?

Anam's Story

Anam, from Manchester in the UK, had always done things 'right' – nourishing her body, honoring her cycle, and living an impressively disciplined life. Yet despite all her hard work and education about her body, she'd struggled to conceive with her husband for more than 18 months, and now, her period had vanished altogether. Deep down, she sensed that her body didn't feel safe. She just couldn't pinpoint why.

Although she was skeptical at first, Anam hesitantly embraced somatic practices. As I got to know her, it became clear that much of her inner turmoil was fueled by anger – a deep-seated resentment stemming from her family's painful rejection of her. Marrying a man outside her religion and culture had been the final straw in a lifetime of disapproval, dismissal, and isolation.

So, in the quiet solitude of her home, Anam embarked on a deliberate, sometimes awkward, journey of releasing this pent-up anger. With each session, the heavy layers of hurt began to peel away. Then, one evening, she felt a deep, pulsing ache in her lower belly – a sign that her period had returned, just five weeks into her daily somatic work. After four healthy cycles, as her body healed and realigned, she received the ultimate gift: she was pregnant.

Once you've made headway in Phase 1 with releasing what's stored, the next step is learning how to track your nervous system state in real time and then respond accordingly.

Phase 2: Regulate to Rewire

You'll no doubt begin to recognize your nervous system state instinctively once you've let go of the past, but below are the key signs to look out for. Use the suggestions for somatic and other tools to help you stay grounded, resilient, and aligned with your inner safety as you navigate the challenges of everyday life.

Dysregulated – Fight-or-Flight and Fawn Response

Sympathetic nervous system activation.

- **Thoughts:** I'm going to fail. Things will fall apart
- **Body:** Tense muscles, racing heart, shallow breath, digestive issues, insomnia
- **Behaviors:** Overworking, snapping at others, starting arguments, or struggling to relax. Fawn may also show up here as a high-alert survival response: over-accommodating, self-abandoning, or prioritizing others' needs to stay safe or avoid conflict
- **Somatic tools:** Any of the practices in Phase 1

Regulated – The 'Just Right' Zone

Regulated nervous system; safe, connected.

- **Thoughts:** The world is a safe place. I'm connected
- **Body:** Deep, slow breaths, relaxed muscles, steady energy
- **Behaviors:** Laughter, connecting with others, clear decision-making
- **Tools to maintain this state:** Expressing your authenticity (see Chapter 17); detox, delegate, and ditch (see Chapter 18); and oxytocin-boosting activities – for example, spending time with friends or having regular orgasms

Dysregulated – Freeze and Collapsed-Fawn Response

Extreme parasympathetic nervous system activation; shutdown, freeze, collapse.

- **Thoughts:** Nothing ever works out for me. There's no point in trying
- **Body:** Heavy limbs, shallow breath, extreme fatigue, brain fog
- **Behaviors:** Withdrawing from others, avoiding tasks, zoning out

- **Somatic tools**: Any of the practices in Phase 1, but done very gently – especially rocking or shaking – so that you wake up the nervous system without overwhelming it. Humming or singing will bring warmth back into the body

Ending the Survival Loop

Learning to recognize your nervous system state and regulate it using the somatic practices in Phase 1 is the gateway to deeper transformation. It prevents new survival patterns from embedding themselves and gives you the emotional stability to begin working at the level of the subconscious (we'll be doing this in the next chapter).

Because now, thanks to the releasing work you've done in Phase 1, you're more *present*. By completing stored stress responses, softening adaptive patterns, and creating space in your nervous system, you've begun to *reclaim your capacity to feel*, and to pay attention to your choices and inner dialogue. And in that space between a stress trigger and your response to it, you gain access to the real roots of your symptoms: the beliefs, identity constructs, and unconscious narratives that have kept you stuck. From that place, you're ready to go deeper.

As you've learned, our subconscious beliefs shape our behaviors – and behind every instinctive reaction is a story our nervous system has learned to tell. This is the friend who never slows down because she believes rest equals laziness. The colleague who over-apologizes because she learned that being disliked wasn't safe. The aunt who spirals into people-pleasing whenever she feels judged. These are adaptive patterns in action built on unprocessed emotional experiences.

A Word of Caution

While somatic practices can be powerful tools for release and healing, deep emotional work – especially when linked to significant trauma – can feel overwhelming for some. If you notice extreme distress, dissociation, or feel unable to regulate on your own, it's essential to seek professional support.

Co-regulation with a trained therapist, somatic practitioner, or trauma-informed professional can provide the stabilization needed to process safely. Everyone's healing journey is unique, and for some, structured guidance is an important part of that process.

Sarah's Story

Sarah is the 24-year-old daughter of immigrant parents who left everything behind in Pakistan to build a better life for her and her brothers in Houston, Texas. She was raised in a conservative Muslim household in which there was an order to things – a way the world should work, a way Sarah should work.

Bullied at school for being different, she quickly learned that blending in was safer than standing out. So, she buried her authentic self-expression and desires and studied to be an accountant, following the logical, stable career path her family wanted for her.

'I felt like I wasn't good enough for anyone,' Sarah told me during our first call. 'I thought I was bothering people just by existing – like they'd be better off if I was quiet. I had abandonment issues, too, so if someone seemed distant, I'd spiral, thinking, What am I doing wrong? *I morphed into whatever version of myself I thought they wanted because I thought they couldn't love the real me. My life was forever winter. That's the best way I can describe it. Dark and depressing.'*

Sarah explained that her health had been unstable since puberty. At 16, she finally had a menstrual cycle, of sorts – sometimes she went 50 or more days between bleeds. Then, at 23, her period vanished completely, and she was diagnosed with PCOS. And while she was extremely dedicated and followed all the conventional advice – cutting out sugar, taking supplements, fixing her gut health, exercising more – nothing was working.

On the day her dad had a heart attack she realized there was something deeper at play. Sitting by his hospital bed, looking at him, Sarah felt nothing. Then, the same thing happened when her best friend passed away. At the funeral, she stood there, numb, aware that she should be crying, that she should be feeling something. But nothing came.

Then, out of the blue, in the fluorescent-lit bathroom of her office, she finally broke. A panic attack gripped her, her body rocking back and forth against the cool tiled wall, her hands gripping her knees. 'I can't do this anymore,' she whispered to herself. That was the moment Sarah decided to reach out to me.

Unsurprisingly, her first big breakthrough came with rocking – the simple, primal rhythm she'd instinctively done during her panic attack. She started practicing somatic work daily with intention, and on the fifth day, she cried 'for the first time in years.'

From there, her healing gathered momentum. After a month of dedicated somatic practice, her nervous system had a new baseline, and she was able to actively acknowledge and challenge the beliefs that had once controlled her when they popped up. Those beliefs that had felt so true – 'I'm not good enough,' 'I'm not lovable' – began to dissolve. She realized that, in fact, she was good enough, lovable, worthy, and deserving.

And then, her period came back. Her cycle quickly settled into 30–35 days, predictable and steady. A year later, she had a perfect 28-day cycle with barely any cramps. No more breast tenderness. No more bloating. And the excess weight she'd been carrying started falling off effortlessly. She was singing, dancing, reading, and drawing again. Her friends all commented on how much happier, lighter, and more alive she seemed. No longer wanting to hide from the world, she chopped off her hair, stopped wearing baggy clothes, and walked into the gym in leggings and a sports bra.

She reapplied to college to follow her dream of becoming a sonographer (ultrasound technician) so she could help other women detect their PCOS and support them through pregnancy. But the most profound shift was in her relationship with her father following his heart attack. Now, they spent precious time together bonding over coffee on the weekends.

'Would you say you're a powerful woman now?' I asked Sarah in our final session. She laughed and said, 'Hell, yes.' Then she paused. 'But really, I just don't care what people think anymore. I don't sit there wondering, Oh no, are they mad at me? *I know I can handle anything now. I feel at peace. Safe.'*

...

Now that you've begun releasing the past from your body, it's time to learn how to rewire the future. In the next chapter, we enter the heart of transforming our subconscious beliefs. Where the beliefs you didn't choose, but have been living by, begin to dissolve.

You'll learn how to reprogram the hidden architecture of your mind and body, so that safety, self-trust, and emotional freedom become your new baseline. This is where the old survival scripts end, and your true story begins.

Chapter 21

ROOT 5: UNCONSCIOUS SAFETY

*'Until you make the unconscious conscious, it
will direct your life, and you'll call it fate.'*

CARL JUNG

Now that you've reconnected with your authenticity, audited your life to create space, begun releasing stored tension from your body, and are working to regulate your nervous system, it's time to rewire the adaptive beliefs that patriarchy planted to keep you small, disconnected, and disempowered. This is where you stop simply breaking from your past and begin breaking from *our* past – the generations of women who had no choice but to shrink themselves to survive.

This chapter will guide you through the process of identifying and rewiring the adaptive beliefs that have shaped your identity and behavior – especially those rooted in generational trauma and patriarchal conditioning.

Some of these adaptive beliefs will dissolve the moment you name them. Others will cling tightly, and some won't even be visible until you've grown beyond them. That's natural. I opened this book with an exploration of our history and biology for a reason: to anchor you in the truth of who you are and who women have always been. When this work challenges you and expands your comfort zone – taking your nervous system into unfamiliar territory – you can return to that truth.

Confronting Our Beliefs and Patterns

Confronting our beliefs is the work of growth and evolution over a lifetime. It unfolds in layers. Different life stages act as mirrors, each one demanding that you challenge your beliefs about who you are and how you've been taught to move through the world.

In your teens, for example, the conditioning often centers around fitting in, being likable, and minimizing discomfort, laying the foundation for people-pleasing, perfectionism, and shame around your body or desires.

Then in your twenties and thirties, those patterns begin to clash with real-life experience. Maybe you burn out from overworking, enter relationships that mirror your old wounds, or realize that your achievements don't make you feel any more worthy. These years often ask you to confront the adaptive belief that your value lies in what you *do*, not who you are.

And when you reach motherhood or caregiving (if it's part of your path) you're cracked open even further. You're confronted with what you inherited unconsciously and asked whether it ends with you. Identity dissolves. Priorities shift. You're forced to reckon with beliefs about sacrifice, control, rest, guilt, and self-abandonment.

Later stages of life – perimenopause, menopause, post-career shifts – can feel like a stripping-away of the roles you've worn for others. Without them, what's left? Here, beliefs about visibility, power, aging, and worth often surface. You may find yourself revisiting old wounds with new wisdom or awakening to truths that were never safe to speak before.

Each chapter of your life holds the invitation to revisit the subconscious programs running the show – and choose differently. And my unique approach to 'rewiring' those programs, ThetaSomatics™, can be used in any life stage.

Cultivating Unconscious Safety

ThetaSomatics draws on neuroscience, somatics, psychology, neuroplasticity, physiology, and a dash of ancient wisdom. Within this method are a range of modalities – breathwork, meditation, and somatic practices – that guide you into deep, embodied transformation. The practice I will share with you shortly is a three-step approach to subconscious rewiring.

You'll then show your subconscious mind that these new authentic beliefs are *safe*, through role models, stories, and representation. And finally, you'll follow a ThetaSomatics Rewiring Practice to normalize expressing these authentic beliefs in your day-to-day reality.

Step 1: Become Aware of Your Adaptive Beliefs

We first explored adaptive beliefs in Chapter 11, when we looked at how we internalize our early experiences as beliefs – many of which are protective, not true. Adaptive beliefs are the unconscious narratives that form when safety is disrupted. Authentic beliefs, meanwhile, reflect who you are when safety is restored.

Create Your 'Reclaiming' List

Below is a set of adaptive (lack of safety) beliefs and their corresponding authentic (safety) beliefs. It's not exhaustive, but it does feature some of the most common and powerful root beliefs seen in therapeutic contexts and research. Use them as a starting point.

When you're ready, read through it and make a list (either by circling them on these pages or writing them in your journal) of the adaptive beliefs that you've noticed you're holding on to *and* the corresponding authentic beliefs that you're ready to 'reclaim.' Yes, these beliefs really are authentic to you, and you can reclaim them. Worthiness, wholeness, and safety formed your original blueprint before you were shaped by the systems, relationships, and environments that taught you to adapt in order to get your needs met.

If you need a reminder of that original truth, spend a moment with a newborn baby or a young child. They don't hustle for their worth. They don't perform to be loved. They simply *are* – whole, worthy, and lovable by nature. That was once you, too. And that version of you still lives within.

Tune in to Your Body as You Read

Although this might seem like an intellectual exercise of the conscious mind – reading through a set of beliefs and identifying which ones resonate – in reality, you're working with both the conscious and subconscious mind simultaneously by tuning in to how your body *responds* as you read. This is what we call *somatic awareness*: using physical sensations as a bridge to deeper truths (remember that your subconscious is part of your nervous system). Your task here is not to analyze but to observe.

Notice what sensations arise in your body as you read – a tightness in your chest, heat in your face, a sudden deep exhale, a twinge in your stomach, or even an urge to skip past certain phrases. These are signals revealing what your subconscious was wired to believe – not what is ultimately true.

Adaptive Beliefs (Lack of Safety)	Authentic Beliefs (Safety)
Wounds of Worthiness	
I don't deserve love.	I'm worthy of unconditional love.
I'm a bad person.	I'm loving and good at my core.
I'm broken.	I'm whole, healing, and wise.
I'm terrible.	I'm human and doing my best.
I'm worthless.	I have inherent worth; I matter.
I'm shameful.	I'm honorable and deserving of respect.
(Part of me believes) I shouldn't be here.	I deserve to live fully and joyfully.
I'm not lovable.	I'm lovable just as I am.
I'm not good enough.	I'm enough and I always have been.
I'm a disappointment.	I'm enough just as I am.

Adaptive Beliefs (Lack of Safety)	Authentic Beliefs (Safety)
I'm insignificant (unimportant).	I'm important; my voice and presence matter.
I don't deserve…	I deserve whatever I desire; I'm inherently worthy.
I deserve only bad things.	I deserve to receive good things.
I'm stupid (not smart enough).	I'm intelligent and always evolving.
Body and Beauty Beliefs	
I'm ugly/my body is hateful.	My body is intelligent, beautiful, and wise.
My body is broken.	My body is wise, responsive, and always on my side.
I'm permanently damaged.	I'm healing; my body and spirit remember how to self-repair.
Guilt Scripts	
I should have done something.	I did the best I could at the time.
I did something wrong.	I'm allowed to learn, grow, and evolve.
I should have known better.	I know better now.
I deserve to be miserable.	I deserve to feel joy, ease, and pleasure.
Emotion and Expression	
It's not okay to feel (show) my emotions.	It's safe to express my emotions; it's safe to take up emotional space.
I can't let it out.	I can choose to release what no longer serves me.
I can't stand up for myself.	I can voice my needs and take up space.
Relational Ruptures	
I can't be trusted.	I can trust myself and my intentions.
I can't trust myself.	I'm learning to trust myself deeply.
I'm different (don't belong).	I belong to my body and this world.
I can't trust my judgment.	My judgment is wise.
I can't trust anyone.	I'm discerning; I choose who to trust.

Adaptive Beliefs (Lack of Safety)	Authentic Beliefs (Safety)
Power and Protection	
I'm in danger.	I'm safe in this moment.
I can't protect myself.	I can learn how to protect and advocate for myself.
I'm not in control.	I have choice and agency.
I'm powerless (helpless).	I'm powerful and can choose differently.
Capacity and Resilience	
I'm weak.	I'm strong; I've always been strong.
I can't get what I want.	I can get what I desire; I deserve to get what I desire.
I'm a failure (will fail).	I can succeed on my own terms.
I can't succeed.	I'm capable of creating what I desire.
I have to be perfect (to please everyone).	It's safe to be imperfect, honest, and free.
I can't stand it.	I can meet challenges with resilience.
I'm inadequate.	I'm more than capable; I'm ready.

Review Your List of Beliefs

Now look through the list of adaptive beliefs you've identified as your own. Take a moment to reflect and connect the dots between those beliefs and the behavioral or relational patterns you noted when you completed your safety self-assessment in Chapter 8.

What you once viewed as personality traits or habits can now be understood as adaptations rooted in a nervous system that didn't feel safe. Once you become aware that you've been operating from a place of survival – how beliefs like 'I don't deserve love' or 'I have to be perfect' shape your reactions, relationships, and sense of self – it becomes easier to see how deeply those beliefs have shaped your daily life and health.

Your subconscious is wired to keep those beliefs alive – not to punish you, but to protect you. It does this by filtering your reality through them. The conversations you engage in, the media you consume, even the song lyrics that stick in your head, they all become reinforcement loops. The belief becomes like a pair of glasses you didn't know you were wearing, coloring how you interpret everything around you.

Your brain's job is to seek evidence that confirms what it already believes. It's not trying to deceive you – it's trying to keep you consistent. But the moment you become aware of this, you have a choice. Ask yourself: *Do I truly believe this 100 percent? Am I really unlovable? Am I actually a bad person?* If even a part of you says 'no,' that's your opening. This is where you ask: *What would I rather believe instead?*

Choose One Adaptive Belief to Shift

From here, you can begin the process of gently rewiring your internal landscape – strengthening a new, authentic belief that reflects who you truly are, not who you had to become in order to cope. Pick something that feels especially present in your life right now – such as shifting 'I'm a failure (will fail)' into 'I can succeed on my own terms.' Or, if you'd rather ease in gently, start with a belief that feels a little less emotionally charged for you. The key is just to begin.

Step 2: Show Your Subconscious That Your Authentic Beliefs Are Safe

Now you're going to continue the process of replacing your chosen adaptive belief with its corresponding authentic belief by sending a powerful message about safety to your subconscious. Here's how to create a new normal for the authentic belief you're reclaiming.

- Find role models. Follow people on social media, watch TED Talks, listen to interviews, and read books by those who embody that authentic belief, or have overcome the adaptive belief you're trying to shift.

- Find a mentor, invest in a life coach, or join a supportive community.

- Seek stories you can come back to you when you need evidence. For example, if you struggle with the adaptive belief 'I'm inadequate,' make a list of people who once doubted their capabilities or intellect but went on to achieve incredible things. Or, if you're working on your self-worth, then a women's circle, gym community, in-person events, or business masterminds can all be great resources for stories of transformation.

Why is this step so important? Because you're shaped by the company you keep. Your subconscious is always absorbing cues, not simply from what people say, but from the behavior and actions they model.[1] This is where we return to the power of mirror neurons – brain cells that fire both when you witness someone performing an action and when you then do it yourself. In other words, your brain doesn't just observe behavior, it begins to internally simulate it.

One of the fastest ways to wire-in a new belief is to surround yourself with people who already embody it. Whether it's in person or through the content or media you consume, consistent exposure to those who live and express your authentic belief sends a powerful message to your subconscious: This isn't just possible – it's normal, safe, and available to you too.

For example, research found that girls studying science, technology, and mathematics who had female mentors were significantly more likely to stay in the field and thrive in male-dominated industries. Those without female mentorship, meanwhile, often experienced a decline in confidence as they progressed through college and into their careers.[2] Why? Because representation reprograms possibility.

And neuroscience shows that we actually model ourselves on those around us – people in our close environment quite literally become part of our internal landscape. When you choose your influences consciously, you're not just changing your mindset, you're rewiring your identity.

Essi's Story

As a competitive swimmer in Finland, Essi carried the relentless drive for perfection from a young age – always striving to improve her times and perform flawlessly. At 22, she moved to Sydney, Australia, to build a new life, and though her competition days were behind her, she continued her disciplined exercise and nutrition routine.

By 30, however, Essi felt profoundly numb. Though outwardly put-together, inside she was untethered, anxious, and exhausted. Retail work paid the bills but left her uninspired, and debilitating migraines became a constant companion. Doctors offered little real help for those, prescribing everything from antidepressants to epilepsy medications. When none of them worked, they simply told her to 'live with it.'

But it wasn't just migraines Essi was suffering with. She didn't understand much about her cycle, but she recognized that her periods weren't even close to regular. And every morning her heart would pound as she grappled with nagging questions like: Who am I? What do I truly love? *She'd completely lost touch with herself.*

Essi was clearly carrying a lot, but after she came to me, it didn't take long for somatic work to take effect. She felt her heart crack open – tears flowed, and astonishingly, her migraines disappeared. For the first time in five years, she experienced a full month free from migraines, and her erratic menstrual cycle began to fall into a natural rhythm.

She felt lighter, liberated, ecstatic. As she explored her adaptive beliefs, she realized that her migraines weren't just physical – they were a clear byproduct of a deeper emotional weight. The belief that she had to be perfect to be loved had shaped her entire way of being, fueling chronic stress and emotional suppression.

Every time she'd feared failure or felt 'behind in life,' her body had absorbed the pressure, storing it as tension and pain. Hypervigilant and disconnected from her true self, she'd unknowingly been carrying years of shame, and now, for the first time, she could finally begin to release it.

Essi began to feel much safer saying yes to new experiences, even when she knew she wouldn't be great at them. She let herself try, fail, and most importantly, enjoy the process – choosing herself and her joy again. She was being silly, fun, and spontaneous; processing difficult emotions when they arose. When the time came for her to start the unconscious safety work outlined in this chapter, she began to reclaim her authentic truth: She didn't need to be perfect. And after a few months, she gained the capacity to do something truly transformative: She changed careers.

For years, her perfectionism and low self-worth had convinced her that she wasn't good enough to be a swimming coach, despite the sport being a core part of her identity. But now she was ready to take the leap. She earned her certification and became a squad coach for 10- to 12-year-olds. Suddenly, she was waking up excited again. Her energy returned. She felt present in her own life.

For the first time since she was a little girl, she wasn't paralyzed by uncertainty or driven by fear. Instead, she felt a deep, unshakable trust in herself. Today, on the rare occasion her migraines return, she knows it's a sign that she's pushing too hard, slipping back into old patterns of perfectionism and self-pressure. So, she slows down, rests, and turns to the ThetaSomatics practices that brought her back to herself in the first place.

'I'm just enjoying my life, and I know I'm going to be okay, no matter what happens,' Essi said in our last session together, a smile radiating genuine belief in her own strength. I asked her, 'Would you confidently say that you're a powerful woman? That you've reconnected with your power?' She didn't hesitate: 'Absolutely. Physically and mentally – both.'

Let's now move to the final, crucial, part of cultivating unconscious safety and claiming your new identity.

Step 3: ThetaSomatics Rewiring Practice

This practice helps your nervous system and subconscious mind *live* the truth of the authentic belief you're reclaiming so that your transformation becomes a felt experience. By harnessing the power of neuroplasticity (the brain's ability to reorganize and rewire itself, and create new neural pathways), it gently rewires old adaptive patterns and beliefs, and teaches your body and mind that this new, authentic way of being and showing up in the world is safe now.

Here are a few things to know before you get started.

Why Does This Practice Work?

To rewire, women need to *move*. We need to feel in our bodies that it's safe to embody and express these new identities after years, decades, or a lifetime of living in contraction. So, the rewiring practice uses a combination of movement, visualization, music, and rhythmic motion to activate key shifts in the brain's chemistry – releasing endorphins, dopamine, and oxytocin, regulating stress, and enhancing your confidence.

Movement itself is one of the fastest ways to create and reinforce new neural pathways because it engages the whole nervous system, not just the brain. It can shift you into a rhythmic, trance-like state that's often linked to theta brainwaves, where your subconscious is more open to change and integration. Dance, in particular, activates multiple brain regions simultaneously, including those that improve neuroplasticity.[3]

The more you move, express, and embody a new, authentic belief, the more natural and automatic it becomes. This isn't just about believing differently – it's about moving and feeling differently; about normalizing and familiarizing a new identity in your nervous system.

How Long Will It Take to Rewire a Belief?

Sometimes, rewiring can happen quickly – especially if you've already immersed yourself in the worlds of your new role models (see above) or if your nervous system feels safe enough to shift. Other times, it takes consistency. That's because neuroplasticity is most responsive to two things: *emotional intensity* (you must *feel* the shift) and *repetition* (you must *repeat* the new pattern enough times for it to stick).

Think of it as like carving a new path through a forest. The more often you walk it, and the more emotionally meaningful it feels, the deeper and more automatic that path becomes. Over time, the old belief is no longer the default pathway because you stopped traveling down that route. Instead, you've been following the path that's aligned with who you really are.

How Often Should I Do This Practice?

I recommend doing it at least three times a week, first thing in the morning (or more often if you feel called). This frequency gives your subconscious enough consistent exposure to start laying down new neural pathways. The goal here isn't perfection, it's momentum. You're signaling to your nervous system, again and again, that this new belief is safe, familiar, and true.

How to Rewire Your Belief

This practice begins with grounding music and movement to regulate the nervous system and open the door to the subconscious mind. It then moves into guided somatic expression to shift old beliefs at a subconscious and nervous system level.

You'll do this by embodying two characters: The version of you shaped by the old, adaptive belief – for example, 'I'm a failure (will fail)' – and the version of you who is living from your authentic truth – for example, 'I can succeed on my own terms.' Moving as these characters helps your body *feel* the difference between adaptive survival patterns and authentic self-worth, allowing you to release the energy of the old belief and anchor the new one in your body.

Adjust the suggested duration of each stage according to your capacity. Just keep in mind that it can take 10 to 15 minutes for your brain to shift into deeper states like theta, especially later in the day. That's why I recommend doing this first thing in the morning, when your brain is already primed for slower, more receptive brainwaves.

Pick Your Playlist

First, choose a space where you won't be disturbed and where you'll feel free to move without inhibition. Now pick a genre of music that matches the energy of the authentic belief you're reclaiming. However, be sure to choose gentle instrumental tracks only, because music without words allows you to stay present in the body and tap into deeper emotional states. For example, if you're reclaiming the belief 'I can succeed on my own terms,' you might want to search for music that feels expansive and uplifting.

Sound is one of the most powerful ways to access the subconscious. The right music creates an emotional atmosphere that softens the nervous system and quietens the analytical mind. This makes it easier to enter a meditative, receptive state, similar to hypnosis, where real subconscious change can begin. Don't overthink it: A simple binaural beats or meditation playlist on YouTube is more than enough.

Drop into Your Body

Press 'play' on the music and take deep breaths in through your nose and out through your mouth to anchor into the present moment. Close your eyes and start the practice by shaking out any tension or tightness. Roll your shoulders and make sure your jaw is unclenched.

Speaking to your body through the language of movement and breath will help you shift out of your thinking mind and into felt awareness – the place where true rewiring begins. Let the music guide you into a deeper state of presence and openness.

Duration: 2–5 minutes

Move Through Resistance

When you feel more centered, you can return your breath to its natural flow and begin making small movements – gentle swaying side to side, hip circles, shoulder rolls – allowing your body to find its own rhythm to the music and letting go of any resistance.

Duration: 2–5 minutes

Express Your Adaptive Belief

Now that your body is present and primed, it's time to bring the old, adaptive belief to life and release the emotional charge. Gently call forward the version of you who believes the adaptive belief – for example, 'I'm a failure (will fail).'

Begin to embody her now. Try her on like a character you're acting out on stage.

- How does she hold herself? Does she shrink, fidget, stay small? Curl into a ball on the floor?
- Does her chest collapse? Does her gaze fall?
- Let your posture reflect the belief as you move around your space.

Then, let her speak. What's her truth? What's she afraid of? Maybe she says:

> 'Nothing ever works out for me.'

> 'Why bother – I'll mess it up anyway.'

> 'No matter how hard I try, it's never enough.'

> 'I'm not the kind of person who succeeds.'

Duration: 2–5 minutes

When she's fully expressed herself and let it all out, take a deep breath and begin to shake her off. Shake your wrists. Shake your hips. Let her energy soften, dissolve. Tell your system: 'We're safe to move forward.'

Duration: 30 seconds–1 minute

Express Your Authentic Belief

Now, try on the authentic character. The version of you who fully owns the authentic belief that corresponds with the adaptive one: 'I can succeed on my own terms.'

- How does this version of you move? With confidence? Softness? Does she stand taller? Take up more space?

- Now move *as her*. Try her on like a character and fully embody her.

- How does she enter a room? How does she take up space without apology? How does she rest into her body, knowing she doesn't have to earn anything?

- Feel what she feels. Feel the joy, the confidence, the freedom. You're not becoming someone else here. You're remembering who you've always been beneath the fear.

- Let your arms, hips, and feet explore new ways of taking up space.

Now speak as her. What does she know? What's her truth? Maybe she says:

'I get to define what success looks like for me.'

'My path may be unconventional, but it's powerful.'

'My way works because it honors who I am.'

Duration: 2–5 minutes

Take Guidance from Your Authentic Self

Now that you've moved into the frequency of your authentic self, let her speak to the version of you who still carries the adaptive belief. Begin speaking out loud – or whisper gently inside your mind. Let her words come through as guidance, compassion, and truth.

- What does your authentic self want your adaptive self to know?
- What does she want to say to the version of you that still feels small, afraid, or not enough?
- What wisdom does she carry that the younger, protective part hasn't been able to hear until now?

Maybe she says:

> 'Your fear is valid, but it's based on someone else's version of success. Not your own.'

> 'Success isn't about doing it perfectly. It's about doing it from your truth.'

> 'We are safe now. You can rest.'

Now expand her focus outward. Let her speak to your life, your relationships, your habits and your choices.

- What would she say to others?
- What routines or roles would she shift?
- What boundaries would she hold?
- How would she show up differently in the spaces you inhabit?

Duration: 2–5 minutes (or for as long as you like)

Integration

When you feel ready to close the practice, slow down gradually, perhaps returning to a gentle sway or placing your hands over your heart and belly. Notice the sensations in your body. Do you feel lighter? More grounded? When you're ready, gently open your eyes and let your gaze land softly. Stay connected to your breath and body.

If it feels right, in your journal write down any insights, emotions, or shifts that came up. How do you feel different from when you started?

Duration: 2-5 minutes

Daily Practice: Act from Your Authentic Belief

This is where the authentic belief starts becoming real in your everyday life. Now that you've felt it in your body through movement, sensation, sound, and visualization, it's time to live it. This step is about *reinforcement*.

The more your subconscious sees you acting from this belief, the more it accepts it as true. Think of it as like muscle memory: Every time you take an action aligned with your belief, you're strengthening the neural pathway in your brain. Over time, it becomes automatic.

Choose one small action today that reflects your new belief. It doesn't have to be big – it just has to be different. Something that slightly disrupts your old pattern and moves you closer to your authentic self. Here are some examples:

- If you're reclaiming the belief 'I'm worthy exactly as I am,' maybe you can speak up in a meeting or post a photo without editing it.

- If your belief is 'I can get what I want,' maybe you can pitch an idea, ask for help, or take the first step toward something you've been putting off.

- If you're rewiring 'It's safe to rest,' you might decline an invitation without guilt or take a nap without justifying it.

And when your nervous system starts to protest (remember, it wants to keep you in the familiar), use your somatic tools to support it. Rock. Breathe. Move. Remember, resistance doesn't mean you're going backward – it means you're rewiring and expanding. You're creating a new comfort zone, and that comes with growing pains.

How to Recognize Signs of Rewiring

Keep going with this practice until you begin to feel a shift in your adaptive belief – whether that's in your body, your thoughts, your behavior, or your emotional reactions (see below). Trust the process. Your consistency is the most powerful ingredient.

Signs You're Making Progress

Awareness: You have a longer pause time between a stress trigger and moving through the survival loop (*see page 125*). You can recognize what's happening and why it's happening. And even though you weren't quite ready to prevent yourself from moving through the rest of the loop, you've made progress.

Action: You recognize what's happening and are able to take steps to avoid the loop: for example, taking deep breaths or a quick walk, listening to music, talking to a trusted friend, or other nervous system regulation techniques that work for you.

Signs You've Reclaimed Your Belief

You feel a sense of safety and relief: This can look like a letting-go feeling – maybe a big sigh, tears, laughter, or as if your heart has opened up a little more. Something feels different! Ninety-nine percent of us won't rewire completely the first time we do this practice, especially when we're dealing with a deeply ingrained belief, trauma, or a memory that we've spent years reinforcing. Remember, repetition plus emotional intensity are the key to creating new neural pathways in the brain and rewiring the nervous system. Keep going – *this works*.

You show up as this belief with confidence: You no longer need to force it or overthink it. You just *are* this person now. You know you don't have to be perfect to be loved.

Your nervous system stays regulated in situations that used to activate you: The things that once sent you spiraling now feel... manageable. You might still experience stress, but it moves through you rather than taking over. You recover faster and take action from your authentic belief.

Let's end this chapter with a story that illustrates the power of subconscious rewiring.

Emily's Story

For Emily, from Denver, Colorado, life had always been a constant push and pull – wanting more but staying stuck, knowing better but falling into the same patterns. At 34, she was living with PCOS, pre-diabetes, knee issues, and depression; she was also numbing with marijuana and alcohol, and carrying far more weight than she was comfortable with.

For years, she'd tried to force *change – 10 years of therapy, thousands of dollars spent on top specialists, all the right books, all the right podcasts. Yet her body, her emotions, and her relationships all felt like a loop she couldn't break.*

The therapy had helped Emily understand intellectually why she was the way she was. She believed her parents' divorce, when she was eight, was the defining moment of her childhood. Raised by her father, she'd learned to take care of herself, to be independent. But she'd also learned how to abandon herself. It showed up in her relationships, where she kept choosing emotionally unavailable men. They weren't bad people, but they were always lacking something she convinced herself she could provide.

Still, something felt missing from her story. So, we did a one-to-one ThetaSomatics™ hypnotherapy session and what surfaced in her subconscious mind changed everything. A memory, long buried, revealed that her mother, an alcoholic, had attempted suicide – and blamed Emily for it. In that moment, as a child, Emily had internalized a belief that had ruled her life ever since: 'I'm responsible for everyone around me.' It was an unbearable emotional and psychological weight to carry.

After the session, Emily finally understood why she could never fully relax, why she was always so focused on fixing everyone around her and always anticipating something going wrong. From that moment, everything started to shift. She completed a ThetaSomatics™ Rewiring Practice every day to reclaim the belief 'I'm not responsible for anyone else,' and began redirecting her energy from controlling everything around her to tuning in to what was happening inside of her.

She started using somatic tools in real time to regulate her nervous system. When difficult emotions built up in her body, she knew how to release them. When a friend's behavior triggered her, she worked through it instead of shutting down. When she sat in traffic and felt anxiety creeping in, she used progressive muscle relaxation and felt her body exhale. She was building something she'd never had before: self-trust.

And then, Emily's new belief was tested when one third of the employees in her company were let go. Suddenly, she was elevated to a leadership position and was asked to share her thoughts and opinions. A year earlier, she would have crumbled under the pressure. But now she handled it with confidence and clarity, taking on her new workload while maintaining strong boundaries and negotiating a significant pay increase.

She started dating again – and this time she was choosing men who met her, who matched her. She started creative writing again, just for the joy of it. She was finally sticking to her habits and routines, and she began making space in her life. At our final session, I barely recognized the woman in front of me. She was sober. Glowing. Her periods were regular. Her pre-diabetes was *nearly fully reversed. Her body felt stronger, looser, and more flexible than ever. Weight was starting to fall off. 'I used to think healing was a finish line,' she told me. 'Like, once I crossed it, I'd be done. But it's not. It's just knowing that no matter what happens, I'll be okay. Because I can handle anything.'*

• • •

This ThetaSomatics rewiring work isn't about fixing you – because you were never broken to begin with – it's simply about remembering who you've always been and giving your body and mind the safety it needs to fully live from and express that truth.

CONCLUSION

'The future is not something we enter. The future is something we create.'

LEONARD SWEET

We've been taught that the feminine is soft, accommodating, endlessly nurturing. But in the cultures that once honored the sacred feminine and the Goddess, she was never just gentle. She was the creator and the destroyer. The force that rose when life was threatened. She held the full spectrum of power: life, death, intuition, rage, creation, boundaries. She wasn't meant to be managed or made palatable. She was meant to be respected.

That's what we've lost, and it's what we're reclaiming now. Because this kind of power – embodied, unapologetic, wild, rooted in truth – doesn't belong in systems built on control, extraction, and suppression. That's why it's been distorted, dismissed, and erased. But it's still here. It's in you. It always was.

Earlier in the book, we explored how women act as an indicator species – our bodies manifesting the tension, distortion, and toxicity of a culture that's lost its way. But when a woman begins to prune away the roots of depletion and nourish those that sustain her, she no longer exists as a warning sign. She becomes a living blueprint for what's possible.

By simply embodying her power, she becomes the initiator of a new reality. She becomes the architect of new systems, new rhythms, and new ways of relating to her body, to others, to the Earth and power itself. She no longer waits for change – she *becomes* it. Not through exhaustion or overcompensation, but through deep nourishment. By no longer abandoning herself. By choosing wholeness over performance. By remembering that her body isn't a problem to be solved but a source of truth to be followed.

Like the Mother Tree, your presence alone nourishes the field.
Your healing creates space for others to grow.

That's how the forest regenerates – through quiet coherence beneath the surface. Feminine leadership operates the same way. Your nervous system becomes the new paradigm. Your presence becomes the pattern-breaker. You walk into a room and the energy shifts – not because you're performing but because you're *rooted* in something real. This is how change begins – not from the top down, but from the inside out.

Walking the Path of Inner Safety

Let the information, techniques, and practices I've shared meet you where you are. Healing isn't a straight line – it's seasonal and cyclical. This book is the next chapter in your lifetime's journey of growth and evolution. A return to yourself and the deeper intelligence inside you – one that doesn't punish or shame but guides and reveals.

And although this is a personal and collective path, we're not meant to walk it alone. We need the healthy, sacred masculine too – the steady, protective presence that supports without controlling, holds without silencing, and stands beside instead of above.

Men must feel comfortable to embrace their feminine – the parts of them wired for care, intuition, collaboration, and emotional truth – and redefine their masculine through depth, not dominance. Structure and softness belong together. Both are necessary – in all of us, in all spaces, and all systems – if we are to build a world that truly holds life.

We must all walk the inner path of alignment before we can rebalance the outer world. We must learn to hold polarity without tipping into extremes. To lead with wholeness instead of with wounds. To bring our gifts forward in service, not in competition.

...

Writing this book has changed me. It asked me to live the work I teach more fully, and to meet myself more honestly. It revealed where I was still performing, still people-pleasing, still holding back, still outsourcing my safety and silencing my voice. To finish it, I had to let go of the version of myself I thought I needed to be and return to the one I actually am. More embodied. More myself. And I'm not going back.

If this book has challenged or provoked you, too: good. If it's cracked something open: even better. This means that something in you is remembering. And that's what this work is about.

This isn't the end. It's the beginning. The breakdown is already happening. And the breakthrough starts now. You're not just an indicator of what's broken. You're the initiator of what comes next.

This is the power you hold.

REFERENCES

Introduction

1. Goldberg E. (2020), 'Mothers Are the "Shock Absorbers" of Our Society': www.nytimes.com/2020/10/14/parenting/working-moms-job-loss-coronavirus.html [Accessed May 15, 2025]
2. Centers for Disease Control and Prevention (2025), 'Suicide data and statistics': www.cdc.gov/suicide/facts/data.html [Accessed May 15, 2025]
3. Levine, H. et al. (2017), 'Temporal trends in sperm counts: a systemic review and meta-regression analysis', *Human Reproduction Update*, 23(6): 646–59.

Chapter 1: Rediscovering Lost Wisdom

1. Montagu, A. (1999), *The Natural Superiority of Women*. Edinburgh: AltaMira Press, p.91.
2. Anxiety & Depression Association of America (ADAA), 'Women and Depression': https://adaa.org/find-help-for-women/depression [Accessed May 15, 2025]
3. Champion Health, 'The Workplace Health Report 2023': https://reba.global/resource/champion-health-the-workplace-health-report-2023.html [Accessed May 15, 2025]
4. Zeng L.N. et al. (2020), 'Gender Difference in the Prevalence of Insomnia: A Meta-Analysis of Observational Studies', *Frontiers in Psychiatry*, 11: 577429.
5. Heades, R. (2023), 'Why are stress levels among women 50 percent higher than men?', Priory Group: www.priorygroup.com/blog/why-are-stress-levels-among-women-50-higher-than-men [Accessed May 15, 2025]
6. National Institutes of Health (2024), 'Autoimmune Diseases', *National Institute of Allergy and Infectious Diseases*: www.niaid.nih.gov/diseases-conditions/autoimmune-diseases [Accessed May 15, 2025]
7. Gao Y. et al. (2023), 'Study of burden in polycystic ovary syndrome at global, regional, and national levels from 1990 to 2019', *Healthcare*, 11(4): 562.

8. Australian Institute of Health and Welfare (2023), 'Endometriosis in Australia 2023': www.aihw.gov.au/reports/chronic-disease/endometriosis [Accessed May 15, 2025]

9. Borumandnia, N. et al. (2021), 'Assessing the Trend of Infertility Rate in 198 Countries and Territories in Last Decades', *Iran Journal of Public Health*, 50(8): 1735–7.

10. Sole-Smith, V. (2019), 'Why Are Girls Getting Their Periods So Young?': www.scientificamerican.com/article/why-are-girls-getting-their-periods-so-young [Accessed May 15, 2025]

11. Alvarez, P. (2022), 'What does the global decline of the fertility rate look like?': www.weforum.org/stories/2022/06/global-decline-of-fertility-rates-visualised [Accessed May 15, 2025]

12. Eichenauer, H. and Ehlert, U. (2023), 'The association between prenatal famine, DNA methylation and mental disorders: a systematic review and meta-analysis', *Clinical Epigenetics*, 15(152).

13. Yehuda R. et al. (2016), 'Holocaust Exposure Induced Intergenerational Effects on FKBP5 Methylation', *Biological Psychiatry*, 80(5): 372–80.

14. Lerner. G, (1994), *The Creation of Feminist Consciousness: From the Middle Ages to Eighteen-seventy*. New York: Oxford University Press USA.

15. Miller, K. (2023), 'Move Over, Men: Women Were Hunters, Too': www.nytimes.com/2023/08/01/science/anthropology-women-hunting.html [Accessed May 15, 2025]

16. Davis, B. and Laffineur, R. (2020), *Neoteros: Studies in Bronze Age Aegean Art and Archaeology in Honor of Professor John G. Younger on the Occasion of his Retirement*. Leuven: Peeters Publishers.

17. Neumann, E. (2015), *The Great Mother: An Analysis of the Archetype*. New Jersey: Princeton University Press, p.95.

18. Holley, P. (2014), 'Creaky joints, sick leave, endless paperwork: ancient Egyptian health care sounds surprisingly familiar', *The Washington Post*: www.washingtonpost.com/news/to-your-health/wp/2014/11/22/creaky-joints-sick-leave-endless-paperwork-ancient-egyptian-health-care-sounds-surprisingly-familiar [Accessed May 15, 2025]

19. Srivastava, M. (2024), 'The Hiranyagarbha Sukta': www.sadhana-sansar.com/post/the-hiranyagarbha-sukta [Accessed May 15, 2025]

20. Shamir, L. (2025), 'The distribution of galaxy rotation in JWST Advanced Deep Extragalactic Survey', *Monthly Notices of the Royal Astronomical Society*, 538(1).

21. Gray, R. (2024), 'Black holes in distant galaxies make them look brighter and bigger': www.thetimes.com/uk/science/article/black-holes-in-distant-galaxies-make-them-look-brighter-and-bigger-bwfof37t3 [Accessed May 15, 2025]

22. Choi, C.Q. (2010), 'Our Universe Was Born in a Black Hole, Theory Says': www.space.com/8293-universe-born-black-hole-theory.html [Accessed May 15, 2025]

23. Friedman, R.E. (1997), *Who Wrote the Bible?* New York: HarperCollins USA, p.235.

24. Merchant, C. (1979), *The Death of Nature: Women, Ecology, and the Scientific Revolution*. San Francisco: Harper & Row, p.145–57.

25. Treber, J. and Thomasson, M.A. (2004), 'From Home to Hospital: The Evolution of Childbirth in the United States, 1927–1940: www.nber.org/system/files/working_papers/w10873/w10873.pdf [Accessed May 15, 2025]

26. Loudon, I. (1986), 'Deaths in Childbed from the Eighteenth Century to 1935': www.cambridge.org/core/services/aop-cambridge-core/content/view/2062B63FD4468574FDB3CD2C1A548241/S0025727300045014a.pdf [Accessed May 15, 2025]

27. Nove, A. et al. (2021), 'Potential impact of midwives in preventing and reducing maternal and neonatal mortality and stillbirths: a Lives Saved Tool modelling study', *The Lancet Global Health*, 9(1): e24–32.

28. MBRRACE-UK, 'Maternal mortality amongst different population groups in England 2020–2022': www.npeu.ox.ac.uk/mbrrace-uk/data-brief/maternal-mortality-2020-2022 [Accessed May 15, 2025]

29. El-Bawab, N. et al. (2023), 'Delayed and denied: Women pushed to the pushed to death's door for abortion care in post-Roe America': www.abcnews.go.com/US/delayed-denied-women-pushed-deaths-door-abortion-care/story?id=105563255 [Accessed May 15, 2025]

30. Kitchener, K. (2025), 'White House Assesses Ways to Persuade Women to Have More Children', Institute for Family Studies: https://ifstudies.org/in-the-news/white-house-assesses-ways-to-persuade-women-to-have-more-children [Accessed May 15, 2025]

Chapter 2: How Patriarchy Shaped Modern Medicine

1. Medical University of Vienna (2024), 'Women live significantly longer in poor health than men': www.meduniwien.ac.at/web/en/about-us/news/2024/news-in-march-2024/women-live-significantly-longer-in-poor-health-than-men-1 [Accessed May 15, 2025]

2. Iacobucci, G. (2024), '"Medical misogyny" leaves many women in pain, MPs' inquiry finds', *BMJ*, 387.

3. Aristotle, translated by Peck, A.L. (1942), *Generation of Animals*. Cambridge, MA: Harvard University Press, pp.27–8.

4. Bornes, L. et al. (2025), 'The oestrous cycle stage affects mammary tumor sensitivity to chemotherapy', *Nature*, 637(8044): 195–204.

5. Yum, S.K. et al. (2019), 'The problem of medicating women like the men: conceptual discussion of menstrual cycle-dependent psychopharmacology', *Translational and Clinical Pharmacology*, 27(4): 127–33.

6. Wang, S. et al. (2024), 'Pan-tissue Transcriptome Analysis Reveals Sex-dimorphic Human Aging': https://elifesciences.org/reviewed-preprints/102449? [Accessed May 15, 2025]

7. He, R. et al (2024), 'Genome-wide single-cell and single-molecule footprinting of transcription factors with deaminase', *PNAS*, 121(52): e2423270121.

8. Rodriguez-Montes, L. et al. (2023), 'Sex-biased gene expression across mammalian organ development and evolution, *Science*, 382(6670).

9. Fillingim, R.B. et al. (1996), 'Sex, gender, and pain: a review of recent clinical and experimental findings', *The Journal of Pain*, 10(5): 447–85.

10. Beery, A.K. and Zucker, I. (2011), 'Sex bias in neuroscience and biomedical research', *Neuroscience Biobehavior Review*, 35(3): 565–72.

11. Phillips, G. et al. (2023), 'Women on the frontline: exploring the gendered experience for Pacific healthcare workers', *The Lancet Regional Health – Western Pacific*, 42: 100961.
12. The Lancet (2024), 'Women in Science: inspiring future generations', *The Lancet Diabetes & Endocrinology*, 12(3): 149.
13. Ross, M.B. et al. (2022), 'Women are credited less in science than men', *Nature*, 608: 135–45.
14. Thompson, J. (2023), 'No one studied menstrual product absorbency realistically – until now': www.scientificamerican.com/article/no-one-studied-menstrual-product-absorbency-realistically-until-now [Accessed May 15, 2025]
15. Vercellini, P. et al. (2013), 'Attractiveness of women with rectovaginal endometriosis: a case-control study', *Fertility and Sterility*, 99(1): 212–8.
16. Maté, G. (2019), *When the Body Says No: The Cost of Hidden Stress*. London: Vermilion, p.58.
17. Skinner, M.K. (2024), 'Epigenetics biomarkers for disease susceptibility and presentative medicine', *Cell Metabolism*, 36(2): 263–77.
18. Marcus, M.D. (2001), 'Psychological correlates of functional hypothalamic amenorrhea', *Fertility and Sterility*, 76(2): 310–16.

Chapter 3: Imposter Syndrome or Imposter Systems?

1. Burki, T. (2024), 'Four industries responsible for millions of deaths each year', *The Lancet Oncology*, 25(7): e285
2. Body and Soul (2024), 'Body + Soul 2024 Sex Census': www.bodyandsoul.com.au/topics/sex-census [Accessed May 15, 2025]
3. Faber, S. (2020), 'The Toxic Twelve: Chemicals and Contaminants in Cosmetics': www.ewg.org/the-toxic-twelve-chemicals-and-contaminants-in-cosmetics [Accessed May 15, 2025]
4. Bagenstose, K. (2023), 'In our blood: how the US allowed toxic chemicals to seep into our lives': www.theguardian.com/environment/2023/sep/13/us-environmental-protection-agency-failed-policy-consumer-chemicals [Accessed May 15, 2025]
5. Faber, S. (2020), 'The Toxic Twelve: Chemicals and Contaminants in Cosmetics': www.ewg.org/the-toxic-twelve-chemicals-and-contaminants-in-cosmetics [Accessed May 15, 2025]
6. Beins, K. et al. (2025), 'Higher hazards persist in personal care products marketed to Black women, report reveals': www.ewg.org/research/higher-hazards-persist-personal-care-products-marketed-black-women-report-reveals [Accessed May 15, 2025]
7. Gore, A. et al. (2024), 'Endocrine Disrupting Chemicals: Threats to Human Health': https://ipen.org/sites/default/files/documents/edc_report-2024-final-compressed.pdf [Accessed May 15, 2025]
8. Spahr, R. (2023), 'Emory-led research first to detect "forever chemicals" in newborns': https://news.emory.edu/stories/2023/09/hs_PFAS_in_newborns_14-09-2023/story.html [Accessed May 15, 2025]
9. Ason, B. (2022), 'Characterization and quantification of endocrine disruptors in female menstrual blood samples', *Toxicology Reports*, 9: 1877–82.

10. Carrington, D. (2024), 'Microplastics found in every human semen sample tested in Chinese study': www.theguardian.com/environment/article/2024/jun/10/microplastics-found-in-every-human-semen-sample-tested-in-chinese-study [Accessed May 15, 2025]
11. Osaka, S. (2024), 'Scientists just figured out how many chemicals enter our bodies from food packaging': www.washingtonpost.com/climate-environment/2024/09/16/more-than-3000-chemicals-food-packaging-have-infiltrated-our-bodies [Accessed May 15, 2025]
12. Yan, Y. et al. (2023), 'The effect of endocrine-disrupting chemicals on placental development', *Frontiers in Endocrinology*, 14: 1059854.
13. Kuta, S. (2025), 'The human brain may contain as much as a spoon's worth of microplastics': www.smithsonianmag.com/smart-news/the-human-brain-may-contain-as-much-as-a-spoons-worth-of-microplastics-new-research-suggests-180985995 [Accessed May 15, 2025]
14. Baker, B.H. et al. (2024), 'Ultra-processed and fast food consumption, exposure to phthalates during pregnancy, and socioeconomic disparities in phthalate exposures', *Environment International*, 183: 108427.
15. Soliman, A. et al. (2014), 'Nutrition and pubertal development', *Indian Journal of Endocrinology and Metabolism*, 18(S1): S39–47.
16. Dougan, M.M. et al. (2024), 'A prospective study of dietary patterns and the incidence of endometriosis diagnosis', *American Journal of Obstetrics and Gynecology*, 231(4): 443.e1–10.
17. Alomran, S. (2023), 'Effect of dietary regimen on the development of polycystic ovary syndrome: a narrative review', *Cureus*, 15(10): e47569.
18. Welch, B.M. et al. (2022), 'Preterm birth more likely with exposure to phthalates': www.nih.gov/news-events/news-releases/preterm-birth-more-likely-exposure-phthalates [Accessed May 15, 2025]
19. *British Medical Journal* (2018), 'Consumption of ultra-processed foods and cancer risk: results from NutriNet-Santé prospective cohort, *BMJ*, 360.

Chapter 4: Women as an Indicator Species

1. Pringle, D. (2022), 'The impact of childhood maltreatment on women's reproductive health, with a focus on symptoms of polycystic ovary syndrome', *Childhood Abuse and Neglect*, 133: 105831.
2. Harris, H.R. et al. (2018), 'Early life abuse and risk of endometriosis', *Human Reproduction*, 33(9): 1657–68.
3. Martins, C. et al (2024), 'Associations between psychological distress in adolescence and menstrual symptoms across life: Longitudinal evidence from the 1970 British Cohort Study': https://pubmed.ncbi.nlm.nih.gov/38494131 [Accessed May 15, 2025]
4. Warwick Business School (2018), 'Are women better investors than men?': www.wbs.ac.uk/news/are-women-better-investors-than-men [Accessed May 15, 2025]
5. Newton-Small, J. (2016), 'How More Women on Wall Street Could Have Prevented the Financial Crisis': https://fortune.com/2016/01/05/wall-street-women-financial-crisis [Accessed May 15, 2025].

6. Weatherford, J. (2011), *The Secret History of the Mongol Queens: How the Daughters of Genghis Khan Rescued His Empire*. New York: Crown.
7. Glubb J.B. (1976), 'The Fate of Empires and Search for Survival', University of North Carolina Wilmington: https://people.uncw.edu/kozloffm/glubb.pdf [Accessed May 15, 2025]
8. Denamur, E. and Matic, I. (2006), 'Evolution of mutation rates in bacteria', *Molecular Biology*, 60(4): 820–7.
9. Moalem, S. and Prince, J. (2007), *Survival of the Sickest: The Surprising Connections Between Disease and Longevity*. London: HarperCollins.
10. Klein, S.L. and Flanagan, K.L. (2016), 'Sex differences in immune responses', *Nature Reviews Immunology*, 16(10): 626–38.
11. Whitacre, C.C. (2001), 'Sex differences in autoimmune disease', *Nature Immunology*, 2(9): 777–80.
12. Shigesi, N., et al. (2025), International Endometriosis Genome Consortium, 'The phenotypic and genetic association between endometriosis and immunological diseases', *Human Reproduction*, 40(6): 1195–209.
13. Hirschberg, A.L. (2020), 'Female hyperandrogenism and elite sport', *Endocrine Connections*, 9(4): R81–92.
14. Lesuis, S.L. (2025), 'Stress disrupts engram ensembles in lateral amygdala to generalize threat memory in mice', *Cell*, 199(1): 121–40.e20.
15. Symphony of Science (2009), 'We Are All Connected' (music video).

Chapter 5: The Biology Lesson That Women Deserve

1. University of Reading (2020), 'Period Pain': www.reading.ac.uk/human-resources/-/media/project/functions/human-resources/documents/factsheet-period-pain-dec2020.pdf [Accessed May 15, 2025]
2. Haakenstad, A. et al. (2022), 'Measuring contraceptive method mix, prevalence, and demand satisfied by age and marital status in 204 countries and territories, 1970–2019: A systematic analysis for the Global Burden of Disease Study 2019', *The Lancet*, 400(10348): 295–327.
3. Palmery, M. (2013), 'Oral contraceptives and changes in nutritional requirements', *European Review for Medical and Pharmacological Sciences*, 17(13): 1804–13.
4. Dolan, E.W. (2025), 'Oxytocin influences moral emotions and decisions, study shows': www.psypost.org/oxytocin-influences-moral-emotions-and-decisions-study-shows [Accessed May 15, 2025]

Chapter 6: A 'Superior' Biological Blueprint

1. Murata, E.M. (2024), 'Circadian rhythms tied to changes in brain morphology in a densely sampled male', *Journal of Neuroscience*, 44(38): e0573242024.
2. Welcome, I.E. (2009), 'Insider: The Female Brain': https://kellercenter.hankamer.baylor.edu/news/story/2009/insider-female-brain [Accessed May 15, 2025]

3. Harvard Health Publishing (2019), 'Marriage and men's health': www.health.harvard.edu/mens-health/marriage-and-mens-health [Accessed May 15, 2025]
4. Jasienska, G. et al. (2006), 'Daughters increase longevity of fathers, but daughters and sons equally reduce longevity of mothers', *American Journal of Human Biology*, 18(3): 422–5
5. Privacy International (2019), 'No body's business but mine: How menstruation apps are sharing your data': https://privacyinternational.org/long-read/3196/no-bodys-business-mine-how-menstruations-apps-are-sharing-your-data [Accessed May 15, 2025]
6. Doctrow, B. (2024), 'Brain changes observed during pregnancy': www.nih.gov/news-events/nih-research-matters/brain-changes-observed-during-pregnancy [Accessed May 15, 2025]
7. Chen, L. et al. (2019), 'The multi-functional roles of menstrual blood-derived stem cells in regenerative medicine', *Stem Cell Research & Therapy*, 10(1).
8. Rodrigues, M.C.O. et al. (2016), 'Menstrual blood-derived stem cells: in vitro and in vivo characterization of functional effects', *Advances in Experimental Medicine and Biology*, 951: 111–21.
9. Meierhenry, J.A. et al. (2015), 'Placenta as a Source of Stem Cells for Regenerative Medicine', *Current Pathobiology Reports*, 3: 9–16.
10. Mosconi, L. (2024), 'Scans show brains' estrogen activity changes during menopause': https://news.weill.cornell.edu/news/2024/06/scans-show-brains-estrogen-activity-changes-during-menopause [Accessed May 15, 2025]

Chapter 7: It's Time for Gender Equality

1. *Financial Times* (2023), 'Gender gaps in economic participation and leadership': www.ft.com/content/17606f25-1d03-4f37-b7f4-f39989af9bde [Accessed May 15, 2025]
2. World Economic Forum (2023), 'Global Gender Gap Report 2023: Gender gaps in the workforce':www.weforum.org/publications/global-gender-gap-report-2023/in-full/gender-gaps-in-the-workforce [Accessed May 15, 2025]
3. Gupta, A.H. (2020), 'Women, Burdened with Unpaid Labor, Bear Brunt of Global Inequality': https://www.nytimes.com/2020/01/23/us/unpaid-work-economy-davos.html [Accessed May 15, 2025]
4. Timmer, J.D. and Woo, D.S. (2023), 'Precarious positions: glass ceilings, glass escalators, and glass cliffs in the superintendency', *Frontiers in Education*, 8.
5. Kahloon, I. (2023), 'What's the Matter with Men?': www.newyorker.com/magazine/2023/01/30/whats-the-matter-with-men [Accessed May 15, 2025]
6. *Financial Times* (2023), 'Gender gaps in economic participation and leadership': www.ft.com/content/17606f25-1d03-4f37-b7f4-f39989af9bde [Accessed May 15, 2025]
7. Joe Rogan Experiences #2255 – Mark Zuckerberg: www.youtube.com/watch?v=7k1ehaEobdU [Accessed May 15, 2025]
8. Masters, R.A. 'True masculine power happens when courage meets vulnerability', *LinkedIn*, www.linkedin.com/posts/robert-augustus-masters-7726354_true-masculine-power-happens-when-courage-activity-7307512039239790592-Y94I [Accessed May 15, 2025]

9. Sabar, A. (2012), 'Update: The Reaction to Karen King's Gospel Discovery': www.smithsonianmag.com/history/update-the-reaction-to-karen-kings-gospel-discovery-84250942 [Accessed July 17, 2025]
10. Watterson, M. (2019), *Mary Magdalene Revealed: The First Apostle, Her Feminist Gospel and the Christianity We Haven't Tried Yet*. New York: Hay House, p.187.

Chapter 8: Introducing the Root Restoration Framework

1. Mate, G. (2022), *The Myth of Normal: Trauma, Illness & Healing in a Toxic Culture*. London: Vermilion, p.337.
2. Ibid.
3. Ibid.

Chapter 9: Stress is More Than What We've Been Told

1. Desborough, J.P. (2000), 'Stress and distress', *British Journal of Anaesthesia*, 85(1): 109–17.
2. Selye, H. (1956), *The Stress of Life*. New York: McGraw–Hill.

Chapter 10: Unlocking the Secrets of the Female Nervous System

1. Wurman, R.S. (1990), *Information Anxiety: What to Do When Information Doesn't Tell You What You Need to Know*. New York: Bantam Bell Publishing Group.
2. VanderPal, G. and Brazie, R. (2024), 'What are gut feelings? Why do they matter?': https://builtin.com/articles/gut-feelings [Accessed May 15, 2025]
3. Sexton, C. (2023), 'Scientists reveal why you should always trust your instincts': www.earth.com/news/trust-your-instincts [Accessed May 15, 2025]
4. Mayer, E.A. et al. (2014), 'Gut Microbes and the Brain: Paradigm Shift in Neuroscience', *Journal of Neuroscience*, 34(46): 15490–6.
5. Bear, T. et al. (2021), 'The microbiome-gut–brain axis and resilience to developing anxiety or depression under stress', *Microorganisms*, 9(4): 723.
6. Pappas, S. (2023), 'What is vagus nerve stimulation for?': www.scientificamerican.com/article/what-is-vagus-nerve-stimulation-for [Accessed May 15, 2025]
7. de Zambotti, et al. (2013), 'Autonomic regulation across phases of the menstrual cycle and sleep stages with premenstrual syndrome and healthy controls', *Psychoneuroendocrinology*, 38(11): 2618–27.
8. Carter, R. et al. (2009), 'Menstrual cycle alters sympathetic neural responses to ortostatic stress in young, eumenorrheic women', *American Journal of Physiology – Endocrinology and Metabolism*, 297(1): e85–91.
9. Prinsen, J. et al. (2025), 'A monthly rhythm of the brain-heart connection': https://www.science.org/doi/10.1126/sciadv.adt1243 [Accessed July 3, 2025]
10. Meng, Y. et al. (2022), 'Menstrual attitude and social cognitive stress influence autonomic nervous system in women with premenstrual syndrome', *Stress*, 25(1): 87–96.

11. Manikandan, S. et al. (2016), 'The role of emotion regulation in the experience of menstrual symptoms and perceived control over anxiety-related events across the menstrual cycle', *Archives of Women's Mental Health*, 19(6): 1109–17.

Chapter 11: The Trauma We Don't See

1. Novotney, A. (2023), 'Women who experience trauma are twice as likely as men to develop PTSD. Here's why': www.apa.org/topics/women-girls/women-trauma?utm [Accessed May 15, 2025]

2. Downey, C. and Crummy, A. (2021), 'The impact of childhood trauma on children's well-being and adult behavior', *European Journal of Trauma & Disassociation*, 6(1): 100237.

3. Creamer, M. et al. (2001), 'Post-traumatic stress disorder: findings from the Australian National Survey of Mental Health and Well-being', *Psychological Medicine*, 31(7): 1237–47.

4. Smith, D.T. et al. (2016), 'Reviewing the assumptions about men's health: an exploration of the gender binary', *American Journal of Men's Health*, 12(1): 78–9.

5. Sadeh, N. et al (2011), 'Gender differences in emotional risk for self- and other-directed violence among externalizing adults', *J Consult Clin Psychol.*, (1): 106–17.

6. Dashorst, P. et al. (2019), 'Intergenerational consequences of the Holocaust on offspring mental health: a systematic review of associated factors and mechanisms', *European Journal of Psychotraumatology*, 10(1): 1654065.

7. Rekor, I. (2024), 'Neurobiological and psychological markers of reaction to extreme stress': www.ean.org/research/resources/neurology-updates/detail/neurobiological-and-psychological-markers-of-reaction-to-extreme-stress-a-three-generation-study-of-holocaust-survivors-and-their-offspring-war-stress-in-ukrainian-refugees [Accessed May 15, 2025]

8. US Department of Veterans Affairs (2016), 'Study finds epigenetic changes in children of Holocaust survivors': www.research.va.gov/currents/1016-3.cfm [Accessed May 15, 2025]

9. Mohn, E. (2024), 'Transgenerational Trauma': www.ebsco.com/research-starters/social-sciences-and-humanities/transgenerational-trauma [Accessed May 15, 2025]

10. Gapp, K. et al. (2018), 'Alterations in sperm long RNA contribute to the epigenetic inheritance of the effects of postnatal trauma', *Molecular Psychiatry*, 25(9): 2162–74.

Chapter 12: Rewiring Our Wounds

1. Clark, C. (2024), 'Could trauma be at the root of autoimmune disease? Dr. Sara Gottfried on the surprising connection': https://camillestyles.com/wellness/autoimmune-disease-and-trauma/?utm [Accessed May 15, 2025]

Chapter 13: The Adaptive Self vs. the Authentic Self

1. Maji, S. (2018), 'Self-silencing and women's health: a review', *International Journal of Social Psychiatry*, 65(1).

2. Morales, J. (2020), 'The heart's electromagnetic field is your superpower': www.psychologytoday.com/us/blog/building-the-habit-of-hero/202011/the-hearts-electromagnetic-field-is-your-superpower [Accessed May 15, 2025]

3. Jakubowski, K.P. et al. (2020), 'The cardiovascular cost of silencing: relationships between self-silencing and carotid atherosclerosis in midlife women', *Annals of Behavioral Medicine*, 56(3): 282–90.
4. Jack, D.C. and Ali, A. (2010), *Silencing the Self Across Cultures: Depression and Gender in the Social World*. Oxford: Oxford University Press.

Chapter 14: Machines Regulate, Humans Feel

1. Pearce, J.M.S. (2002), 'Silas Weir Mitchell and the "rest cure"': https://jnnp.bmj.com/content/75/3/381 [Accessed May 15, 2025]
2. Stetson, C.P. (1892), 'The Yellow Wall-Paper': www.nlm.nih.gov/exhibition/theliteratureofprescription/exhibitionAssets/digitalDocs/The-Yellow-Wall-Paper.pdf [Accessed May 15, 2025]
3. Ekman, P. (1992), 'Facial Expression and Emotion': www.paulekman.com/wp-content/uploads/2013/07/Facial-Expression-And-Emotion1.pdf [Accessed May 15, 2025]
4. Pert, C.B. (1997), *Molecules of Emotion: Why You Feel the Way You Feel*, New York: Prentice Hall and IBD.
5. Elphick, M.R. (2018), 'Evolution of neuropeptide signalling systems', *Journal of Experimental Biology*, 221(3).
6. McEwen, B.S. (2007), 'Physiology and Neurobiology of Stress and Adaptation: Central Role of the Brain', *Physiological Reviews*, 87(3): 873–904.
7. Richter-Levin, G., & Akirav, I. (2003), 'Emotional tagging of memory formation—in the search for neural mechanisms': https://pubmed.ncbi.nlm.nih.gov/14629927 [Accessed July 22, 2025]
8. Salk Institute (2024), 'New tools reveal neuropeptides, not neurotransmitters, encode danger in the brain': www.sciencedaily.com/releases/2024/07/240722155157.htm [Accessed May 15, 2025]
9. Schleip, R. 'Fascia as a sensory organ: Clinical applications': www.fasciaresearch.de/publications/ExcerptTerraRosaSensory.pdf [Accessed May 15, 2025]
10. Michalak, J. et al. (2021), 'Myofascial Tissue and Depression', *Cognitive Therapy and Research*, 46(3): 560–72.
11. Noetel, M. et al. (2024), 'Effect of exercise for depression: systematic review and network meta-analysis of randomised controlled trials', *BMJ*, 384: e075847.
12. Gozalo-Pascual, R. et al. (2023), 'Efficacy of the myofacial approach as a manual therapy technique in patients with clinical anxiety: A randomized controlled clinical trial', *Complementary Therapies in Clinical Practice*, 51: 101753.
13. Phan, V.T. et al. (2021), 'Widespread myofascial dysfunction and sensitisation in women with endometrios-associated chronic pelvic pain: a cross-sectional study', *European Journal of Pain*, 25(4): 831–40.
14. Bürger, Z. et al. (2023), 'Stressor-Specific Sex Differences in Amygdala–Frontal Cortex Connectivity': https://pubmed.ncbi.nlm.nih.gov/36769521 [Accessed July 22, 2025]
15. Stevens, J.S. and Hamann, S. (2012), 'Sex differences in brain activation to emotional stimuli: A meta-analysis of neuroimaging studies', *Neuropsychologia*, 50(7): 1578–93.

Chapter 15: Women – From Indicators to Initiators

1. Simard, S. (2021), *Finding the Mother Tree: Discovering the Wisdom of the Forest.* London: Allen Lane.

Chapter 19: Root 3: Environmental Safety

1. Shukla, A.P. et al. (2015), 'Food order has a significant impact on postprandial glucose and insulin levels', *Diabetes Care,* 38(7): e98–9.
2. Armitage, H. (2018), 'Diabetic-level glucose spikes seen in healthy people': https://med.stanford.edu/news/all-news/2018/07/diabetic-level-glucose-spikes-seen-in-healthy-people.html [accessed May 15, 2025]
3. Brown, P. (2004), 'Fish stocks in danger as males changes sex': www.theguardian.com/environment/2004/jul/10/endangeredspecies.uknews [Accessed May 15, 2025]

Chapter 20: Root 4: Historical Safety

1. Ozaki, M. et al. (2022), 'Effect of the sway bed on autonomic response, emotional responses, and muscle hardness in children with severe motor and intellectual abilities: a pilot study', *Healthcare (Basel),* 10(11): 2337.
2. Cross, R.L. et al. (2017), 'Implementation of rocking chair therapy for veterans in residential substance use disorder treatment', *Journal of the American Psychiatric Nurses Association,* 24(3): 190–8.

Chapter 21: Root 5: Unconscious Safety

1. Hyeonjin, J. and Lee, S.H. (2018), 'From neurons to social beings: short review of the mirror neuron system research and its socio-psychological and psychiatric implications', *Clinical Psychopharmacology and Neuroscience,* 16(1): 18–31.
2. Reynolds, E. (2023), 'Female peer mentors have long-lasting positive impact on female STEM students': www.bps.org.uk/research-digest/female-peer-mentors-have-long-lasting-positive-impact-female-stem-students [Accessed May 15, 2025]
3. Teixeira-Machado, L. et al. (2018), 'Dance for neuroplasticity: A descriptive systemic review', *Neuroscience & Biobehavioral Reviews,* 96: 232–40.

ACKNOWLEDGMENTS

I'm deeply grateful to be alive at a time when it's possible to write a book like this. To speak so openly about how the systems in which we live shape our health, authentic self-expression, and power is something many women before me could not do safely, and in many parts of the world, still can't.

I feel incredibly fortunate to stand on the shoulders of so many women – to speak with them across time, to carry their insights forward, and to weave their wisdom into something new. My life and work have been profoundly shaped by those who came before me. Their scholarship, their activism, and their stories created the conditions for this book to exist. I hope readers explore the references section as a gateway into that wider lineage because no work like this is created in isolation. It's part of a much older conversation – one I'm honored to continue.

I'd like to thank the following people:

Kezia Bayard-White: This was an ambitious project – every chapter could have been a book in itself – and I was afraid I'd be asked to water it down. I needn't have worried. Thank you for helping me find the gold in a very cathartic first draft, and for pushing me to refine without losing the fire. Your brilliance, compassion, and razor-sharp mind made this book infinitely stronger. Working with you was a joy.

Oscar Janson-Smith: You may be my agent, but you gave me agency. Thank you for championing my voice and vision from the very beginning, and for being a steady source of wisdom, clarity, and encouragement.

Debra Wolter: Your grounded presence and editorial precision held me through the most demanding stretch of this process. Thank you for your fearless edits and unwavering clarity. I felt truly supported.

The team at Hay House UK, especially Michelle Pilley, Julie Oughton, and Portia Allen-Chauhan: Thank you for believing in the message of this book and standing behind it with such conviction. Julie and Portia, your care, creativity, and persistence in ensuring that both the cover and internal visuals reflected the heart of this work meant the world to me. I'm so grateful to be in such thoughtful hands.

Mirielle Harper: I'm endlessly thankful that you saw this book in me – long before the idea had entered my mind – and encouraged me to bring it into form. Your early belief lit the match, and I'll never forget it.

Every expert who generously shared their time, knowledge, and voice: Your contributions added depth and a dimension that made this book what it is. Thank you for sharing so generously and openly with me.

Mary Riposta: Our shared journey of self-discovery has been a gift. Your friendship and collaboration have illuminated so much. Thank you for walking beside me.

My clients: Your stories, patterns, and breakthroughs are woven through every page. You have been my greatest teachers.

The women who have shared their stories with me over the years: Your courage, vulnerability, and truth-telling live inside these pages. We heal when we speak to each other. Your stories are part of the collective remembering and have inspired me to keep going.

Jen Kruidbos, Ida Carstedt, and Irina Mozo: I'll be forever grateful we came together at the exact moment I needed the depth of sisterhood most.

You've cracked open my heart, expanded my mind, and held me with radical honesty and unconditional love. Thank you for showing me how potent female friendship truly is. I love you so much and can't wait to keep watching you change the world.

Georgina Capdevila, Ana Gasol, and Concepticó Gasol: Your depth, intuition, and embodied example of womanhood have shaped me more profoundly than words can express. You move through the world with an undeniable power and fierce knowing that has been both a mirror and a guide. You've each been mentors to me in your own way, and I carry your influence with deep reverence.

Mum and Dad: I believe we choose our parents, and I chose exceptionally well. Thank you for never taking no for an answer on my long and winding path to full health – and for your relentless support, your deep love, and your unshakable belief in me.

Thank you for allowing me to share moments from our lives in this book, and for showing me, by example, how to live bravely and with integrity. You gave me a rich education, nourished my voracious appetite for books, and gifted me both wings and roots – the freedom to follow what lit me up, and the safety to walk my own path, even when it took me across the world.

There is no version of this book, or of me, that could exist without the unique blend of both of you. I'm the woman I am because of the home you created, the values you lived, and the wisdom you passed down. I hope this book shows you just how many of your pearls I absorbed and just how deeply grateful I am.

Jasper: I'm so proud to be your sister. Your sharp intellect, humor, and quiet strength have grounded me through so many seasons. I loved watching you become the man you are.

The teachers, librarians, booksellers, and professors who nourished my mind: A special mention to my teachers at Geelong Grammar School in Australia, who taught me to question deeply, think critically, and never settle for surface answers. You gave me permission to be curious, to challenge convention, and to trust that my voice mattered.

To the friends I've lost along the way and whose lives ended far too soon: thank you for reminding me what really matters. You taught me to stop waiting, to say the true thing, to feel it all, take the risk, and to milk every second from this wild, precious life. Harriet and Stanham, I think of you every day.

The brilliant friends, mentors, and colleagues from my time in London's corporate jungle: Thank you for the sharp edges, the lessons, and the proximity to thinkers and scientists whose work echoes through these pages. That chapter of my life shaped me in ways I'm only just beginning to understand.

All those who reminded me I didn't have to do this alone: Thank you for the steadiness, softness, and sanctuary. To Helen, who offered me the quiet of her beach house where the idea for this book finally landed in full at 4 a.m. as the sun rose. To my big, wonderful family who are spread out around the world, especially my aunts Jane and Anna, thank you for checking in and cheering me on. To Wendy and Chris, who have supported me for seven years with such generosity and love. And to Emily Pollock, mentor, big sister, angel. Thank you for arriving exactly when I needed you. Your guidance, presence, and capacity to hold me through some of the most difficult moments of my life changed my trajectory. I will never forget it.

Bijanka Bacic and Katherine Mathews: My chosen sisters. Bijanka, thank you for gently introducing this corporate burnout to the creative process, and for showing me what it means to flow. Kate, thank you for loving every version of me as we grew from girls into women. Your friendship is one of the truest things in my life.

And last, but never least, Andrew: Thank you for creating the kind of safety that made it inevitable I would step into my full power. Your love helped me fall back in love with myself. Realizing how deeply I want to be the mother of your children became a seed of resilience that carried me through some of my hardest days. I couldn't have ushered in my first two babies – this and my previous book – in just eight months without you.

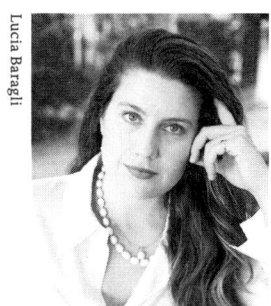
Lucia Baragli

ABOUT THE AUTHOR

Isabella Mainwaring is an author, speaker, and respected voice in hormone science who is devoted to restoring women's health and vitality. Her work bridges hormonal physiology, trauma healing, nervous system regulation, and subconscious reprogramming to help women unravel survival patterns and reclaim authority over their bodies and lives.

After experiencing fertility challenges, PCOS, and corporate burnout as a strategy consultant in London, Isabella retrained in integrative nutrition, functional hormone health, and trauma and PTSD recovery. This led her to create her unique therapeutic method, ThetaSomatics™, which blends brainwave science, somatics, and psychology for deep, lasting transformation.

Through her writing, courses, and ThetaSomatics work, Isabella has supported thousands of women to return to clarity, energy, and full-spectrum expression. Her first book, *Hormone Balance for Dummies*, established her as a trusted authority in the global women's health movement.

Born in London, raised in Australia, and now based in Spain, Isabella is building a worldwide movement of women reclaiming their power.

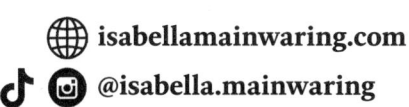

isabellamainwaring.com
@isabella.mainwaring

We hope you enjoyed this Hay House book. If you'd like to receive our online catalogue featuring additional information on Hay House books and products, please contact:

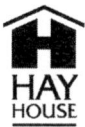

Hay House UK Ltd
1st Floor, Crawford Corner,
91–93 Baker Street, London W1U 6QQ
Tel: +44 (0)20 3927 7290; www.hayhouse.co.uk

Published in the United States of America by:
Hay House LLC
PO Box 5100, Carlsbad, CA 92018-5100
Tel: (760) 431-7695 or (800) 654-5126
www.hayhouse.com

Published in Australia by:
Hay House Australia Publishing Pty Ltd
18/36 Ralph St., Alexandria NSW 2015
Tel: +61 (02) 9669 4299
www.hayhouse.com.au

Published in India by:
Hay House Publishers (India) Pvt Ltd
Muskaan Complex, Plot No. 3,
B-2, Vasant Kunj, New Delhi 110 070
Tel: +91 11 41761620
www.hayhouse.co.in

Let Your Soul Grow

Experience life-changing transformation – one video at a time – with guidance from the world's leading experts.

www.healyourlifeplus.com

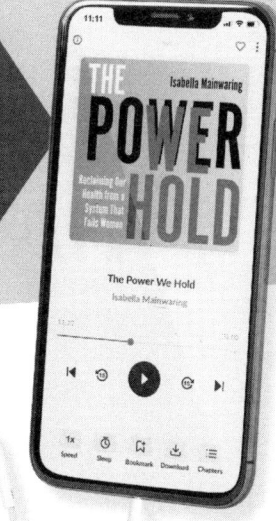

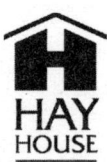

CONNECT WITH
HAY HOUSE
ONLINE

hayhouse.co.uk   @hayhouse

@hayhouseuk   @hayhouseuk.bsky.social

@hayhouseuk   @HayHousePresents

Find out all about our latest books & card decks • Be the first to know about exclusive discounts • Interact with our authors in live broadcasts • Celebrate the cycle of the seasons with us • Watch free videos from your favourite authors • Connect with like-minded souls

'The gateways to wisdom and knowledge are always open.'

Louise Hay